The Chain of Immunology

The Chain of Immunology

GEORGE FEINBERG
MSC, DVM, FIBiol
Visiting Professor, Department of Immunology
St Thomas's Hospital
Medical School, London

MARK A. JACKSON
BSc
Medical Student, St Thomas's Hospital
Medical School, London

BLACKWELL SCIENTIFIC PUBLICATIONS
OXFORD LONDON EDINBURGH
BOSTON MELBOURNE

First published 1983

Photoset by Enset Ltd, Midsomer Norton, Avon
and printed and bound in Great Britain by
Butler & Tanner Ltd, Frome, Somerset

DISTRIBUTORS

USA
 Blackwell Mosby Book Distributors
 11830 Westline Industrial Drive
 St Louis, Missouri 63141

Canada
 Blackwell Mosby Book Distributors
 120 Melford Drive, Scarborough
 Ontario, M1B 2X4

Australia
 Blackwell Scientific Book Distributors
 31 Advantage Road, Highett
 Victoria 3190

British Library
Cataloguing in Publication Data

Feinberg, George
 The chain of immunology.
 I. Immunology
 I. Title   II. Jackson, Mark A.
 616.07'9   QR181

ISBN 0-632-00881-4

Contents

Acknowledgements, vi

Prologue, vii

List of Acronyms and Abbreviations, viii

Introduction, 1

1   The Cell's the Thing, 3

2   Enter the Antigen, 18

3   The Covert Immune Response, 22

4   The Overt Immune Response and
    Immune Reaction, 25

5   Mishaps of Immune Response and
    Immune Reaction, 34

Epilogue, 43

Bibliography, 44

Index, 45

The Chain *inside back cover*

v

Acknowledgements

Pregnancies have a way of overruning their EDD (Expected Date of Delivery), but the gestation period of *The Chain of Immunology* must have set an all-time record. So, I must first acknowledge the forbearance—amounting at times to martyrdom—of Per Saugman of Blackwell Scientific Publications, who never once contemplated terminating the pregnancy.

My next vote of appreciation must go to Professor Dudley Dumonde and to the Trustees of St Thomas's Charitable Trust, whose beneficence in extending my useful professional life was undoubtedly the salvation of the present opus.

Then there is Dr. Betty Sanchez, who never once let me forget my obligation to keep the commitment I had made to produce this book.

And last, but proverbially not least, I owe my thanks to Christine Stafford, who toiled nobly to transcribe manuscript to typescript.

G.F.

Prologue

Is immunology as complex as the immunologist makes it out to be? Perhaps. But viewed through bifocal lenses, focusing respectively on teleology and pragmatism, it is possible to weave a fairly straight path through the jungle of statements and counterstatements, images and mirages, facts and fancies which make up 20th century immunology.

No would-be explorer would plunge into a charted jungle without a route map, together with a few notes on some of the unfamiliar flora and fauna he will encounter on his travels. He would also provide himself with a lexicon and phrase book of the foreign tongues of the regions he will explore.

Perforce, route maps highlight the highways, only sketching in the byways. For the less defined areas and more minute details, should these be of additional interest to him, our explorer would complement his informational sources with specific area maps and the larger guide books. *The Chain of Immunology* is an annotated route map cum lexicon and phrase book, for the would-be explorer of the immunological jungle.

In putting *The Chain* together, I have had to make arbitrary decisions about which were the highways, which the byways, of immunology and define the vocabulary in accordance with my own philological tastes. The result is very much a personal testament of immunology.

As with geographical route maps, my immunological map is not intended to supplant the larger, more detailed treatises and specialized texts on immunology. Rather, it is meant to complement them. Immunology has become so vast and so specialized that no one book can be all things to all immunologists, or to those simply working on the fringes of immunology.

In this respect, I hope it will serve the reader as well as it has, in blackboard and lecture form, served me as a teaching device and my students as a learning aid over the past ten years. It is at the persistent instigation of my students that *The Chain of Immunology* now becomes a book. In fact, it was one of these students, Mark Jackson, whom I am pleased to welcome as co-author, who stimulated and assisted me in getting the book into print; and whose artistic talents have been put to use in providing the free-hand illustrations for the book.

One personal principle has guided me in the writing of *The Chain:* I have never believed that learning has to be deadly dull, or text books swathed in solemnity. Consequently, the reader should recognize some light touches (= divertissements) scattered through the text. If I have attained my objective, he/she will find *The Chain* fun to read: a book to live with, rather than one to languish unloved on the bookshelf.

George Feinberg

N.B: a word to the reader. Immunology is a circuitous subject, constantly anticipating itself in its unfolding. For the sake of brevity and continuity, I have avoided cross-referencing and endless q.v.ing. Therefore, for ease of understanding, the chart and notes should be twice studied conjointly, in rapid succession. The first time round you will prematurely meet words and concepts which are more fully explained later. The second time you meet them they will be old friends; and in this case, familiarity breeds content. Throughout the text italics are used for emphasis or for introduction of a new term; bold type is used where a term is defined. Again for the sake of continuity, a term may not necessarily be defined fully at first meeting, but at a later—more appropriate—encounter. Finally, where a verbal description is given of a structure or event—e.g. an immunoglobulin molecule, the complement barrage—I urge you to attempt a diagrammatic construction with pen and paper. This will fix the matter more firmly in your mind than will any accompanying diagram.

Acronyms and Abbreviations

a.a.	amino acid
Ab	Antibody
Ag	Antigen
ALG	Anti-Lymphocyte Globulin
ALS	Anti-Lymphocyte Serum
ANA	Anti-Nuclear Antibody
ATP	Adenosine TriPhosphate
B-cell	Bursa/Bone marrow derived lymphocyte
BALT	Bronchial-Associated Lymphoid Tissue
BCG	Bacillus Calmette-Guérin
C	Complement
ca.	circa (about)
–C = C–	Carbon = Carbon double bond
C_H/C_L	Constant domains of Heavy and Light chains respectively
cvf	cobra venom factor
DH	Delayed Hypersensitivity
DNA	Deoxyribose Nucleic Acid
DNCB	DiNitroChloroBenzene
ECF-A	Eosinophil Chemotactic Factor of Anaphylaxis
ELISA	Enzyme-Linked ImmunoSorbent Assay
Fab	Fragment antigen-binding
F(ab')$_2$	Fragment of Ig with 2 antigen-binding sites
Fc	Fraction crystallizable
FCA	Freund's Complete Adjuvant
FIA	Freund's Incomplete Adjuvant
GALT	Gut-Associated Lymphoid Tissue
GvH	Graft-versus-Host reaction
H	Heavy Ig chain
HAs	Histocompatibility Antigens
HLA	Human Leucocyte Antigen
5-HT	5-HydroxyTryptamine
IC	IntraCutaneous
ID	IntraDermal
Ig	Immunoglobulin
IM	IntraMuscular
IP	IntraPeritoneal
IR	Immune Response
IRC	Immune ReaCtion
Ir gene	Immune response gene
IV	IntraVenous
KAF	Konglutinin Activating Factor
K cell	Killer cell
L	Light Ig chain
LADs	Lymphocyte Activating Determinants
LATS	Long-Acting Thyroid Stimulator
Ly Ags	nomenclature used to designate mouse T-Lymphocyte surface markers
Leu Ags	nomenclature used to designate surface markers on T-cell Leucocytes in man
MAF	Macrophage Activating Factor
MHC	Major Histocompatibility Complex
MIF	Migration Inhibition Factor
MLR	Mixed Lymphocyte Reaction
Mφ	Macrophage
mRNA	messenger RNA
NCF-A	Neutrophil Chemotactic Factor of Anaphylaxis
NK cell	Natural Killer cell
OKT Ags	arbitrary nomenclature used to designate surface markers on human T-cells
PAF	Platelet Activating Factor
PCA	Passive Cutaneous Anaphylaxis
PG	ProstaGlandin
PPD	Purified Protein Derivative (of tuberculin)
RA	Rheumatoid Arthritis
RBC	Red Blood Cell
Rh	Rhesus blood group antigen
RIA	RadioImmunoAssay
RNA	RiboNucleic Acid
rRNA	ribosomal RNA
SC	Secretory Component
SD Ag	Serologically Determined antigen
SLE	Systemic Lupus Erythematosus
SRF	Skin Reaction Factor
SRS-A	Slow-Reacting Substance of Anaphylaxis
-S-S-	diSulfide bridge
T-cell	Thymus derived lymphocyte
T_{cyt}	cytotoxic T-cell
T_h	helper T-cell
tRNA	transfer RNA
T_s	suppressor T-cell
TSH	Thyroid Stimulating Hormone
V_H/V_L	Variable domains of Heavy and Light chains respectively
WBC	White Blood Cell

Introduction

Immunology? . . . What's that? This is the common reaction of the non-immunologist coming face-to-face with the term immunology. It may also be the reaction of the immunologist faced with the many-sided aspects of immunology.

A tentative definition could be:

Immunology is the science *(logy)* of the vertebrate animal's *recognition* of, *specific response* to and subsequent *memory* of an *antigen,* and the *reaction* between the *products* of that response and the antigen which provoked it; as *originally* conceived, to make the animal exempt **(immune)** from *infection.*

Immune recognition The physiological mechanism by which the animal body recognizes a 'foreign' substance (antigen) as something against which it is capable of making an immune response.

A system of 'bumps' and 'hollows'

On a wider scale, *recognition* is the basis for biological activity: enzymes must recognize their substrates, appropriate cell receptors must recognize hormones, nerve cell receptors must recognize neurotransmitters . . . and the immune system must recognize specific antigens. On the 'shop-floor' level, it all comes down to a system of 'bumps' and 'hollows'. Molecules are three-dimensional structures, with uneven surfaces contorted into an almost infinite variety of projections ('bumps') and indentations ('hollows'). Recognition occurs when the shape of a 'bump' closely corresponds to the form of

a 'hollow'. The one can then fit snugly into the other and allow a number of short-range forces to come into play. These 'bumps' and 'hollows' come under several functional names. Immunologically speaking, we call the 'bump' on an antigen an *epitope.* A *paratope* is the hollow on the antibody which recognizes the epitope. *Receptor* is the name we give 'bumps' or 'hollows' associated with cell membrane proteins: for example, the epitope recognition receptors on T lymphocytes, and immunoglobulin and complement receptors on various leucocytes.

Immune response (IR) The physiological chain of events induced in the vertebrate animal exposed to antigen, leading to certain IR products; IR products may be **humoral** (i.e. production of *antibodies*) or/and **cellular** (i.e. production of *aggressive lymphocytes*); the response after a first exposure to an antigen is called a **primary response,** that to subsequent exposure to the same antigen is called a **secondary response.**

Specificity Aptly described by Ehrlich as a 'key-in-lock' situation in which only the key which fits the lock will open it; hence, a matter of a *good fit* between a 'key' (the *epitope*) on an antigen molecule and a 'lock' (the *paratope*) on an antibody molecule or receptor on a T-cell; in our own terminology, a good fit between an epitope 'bump' and a paratope or receptor 'hollow' (Figure 1).

Memory The quicker recognition of an antigen on second meeting, so that the secondary response is *faster, more intense* and *longer-lasting* than the primary.

Immune reaction (IRC) The interaction between an antigen and the specific IR products provoked by it; may take place **in vivo** (in the living animal) or **in vitro** (literally, 'in glass'); *in vivo* it may produce protection

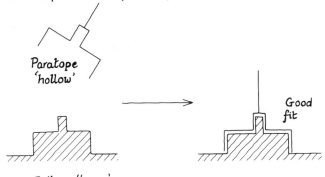

Figure 1.

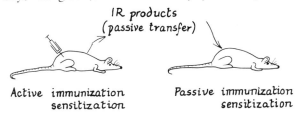

Figure 2.

1

(**immunity**) or, paradoxically, harm (**hypersensitivity**); the product resulting from combination of antigen and antibody is called an **immune complex**.

Immunity The state of possessing IR products to an antigen; may be acquired *actively* through the animal's own response (= **active immunity**), or *passively* through transfer (= **passive transfer**, Figure 2) of antibodies or lymphocytes from an actively immunized animal (= **passive immunity**); the immunized animal *donating* the IR products is termed the **donor**, the *receiving* animal giving *hospitality* to the Ab or activated lymphocytes is called the **recipient** or **host**; active immunity may arise *spontaneously* as the result of infection, or be deliberately **induced** by injection of antigen (**immunization**); teleologically (= with a purposeful end in mind) it is an immune defence mechanism.

Immunization Originally, the induction of protection against infection by administration of a vaccine; now *any administration* of an antigen to induce an IR.

Hypersensitivity A situation in the living animal in which combination of antigen with IR products leads to *inflammation* and cell or tissue damage; may also be *active* or *passive*, *spontaneous* or *induced*.

Sensitization The process of induction of *hypersensitivity* to antigen.

Inflammation Those events which take place in living tissue as a result of certain types of provocation, such as an external agent (physical, chemical, infectious organism), or an IRC; involves *vascular dilatation* and *increased capillary permeability*, resulting in *leakage of plasma* into and *leucocyte infiltration* of the tissue; if severe, may lead to tissue damage and even *necrosis* (= death) of the tissues involved.

The problem of defining two of the basic elements of immunology—antigen and antibody—is like that of defining a snake biting its own tail: neither has demonstrable beginning or end. In the snake analogy, the head is that part holding the tail, the tail is that part being held by the head. In immunology, the antigen is that which induces antibody and antibody is that which is induced by antigen. More scientifically, and acknowledging the fact that the IR has a cellular side as well as an antibody side:

Antigen (Ag) Something which *gen*erates a response against (= *anti*) itself; since the response generated is the *immune* response, alternatively (and perhaps better) termed **immunogen**.

Antibody (Ab) That which an animal makes as a response against some 'foreign' substance *(body)* and which is found circulating in the fluid portion (**humour**) of the blood—hence, a product of the **humoral** IR; Ab has the capacity to bind specifically with its Ag.

Antiserum The fluid portion of clotted blood (*serum*) from an immunized animal, which contains one or more specific *anti*bodies to one or more Ags.

Thus, immunology, as the study of IR and IRC, can be considered a *chain* of events triggered off by Ag: hence, *The Chain of Immunology*. As with chains of the Ab molecule, the immunology chain can be divided into a number of sections (= *domains*), of which one is variable, the rest constant, in nature. Each of the **constant domains** describes a relatively *constant* set of events in the normal IR, whereas in the **variable domain** are found the *inconstantly* occurring immunological mishaps.

Chains are made of links. In the antibody chains the links are a series of amino acids. In the immunology chain the links are those cells, the tissues they make up, and their products, which participate in the IR and IRC. Therefore, *'The Cell's the Thing'* makes up the first domain of *The Chain of Immunology*.

The second domain starts with the arrival of Ag and considers the way it is dealt with—hence, *'Enter the Antigen'*.

When the Ag is processed and the answer comes back 'all systems go', the IR leaps into operation. At the outset, much is going on behind the scenes, with little open evidence of activity. This is followed by a state in which the IR is openly demonstrable in terms of the products of the response and the IRCs between these IR products and Ag. So the third domain is *'The Covert Immune Response'* (*covert* = closed, hidden), while the fourth is *'The Overt Immune Response and Immune Reaction'* (*overt* = open).

But, as in all biological systems, in immunology things do not always go according to Nature's 'grand plan'. Robert Burns, the Scottish poet, phrased it nicely when he wrote: 'The best laid schemes o' mice and men gang aft a-gley.' And so we must add to the immunology chain a final domain: *'Mishaps of Immune Response and Immune Reaction'*, in which we consider some of the things which can go wrong.

1. The Cell's the Thing

Immunology, like the Bible itself, must begin with 'genesis': 'In the beginning . . .'.

Just as in the Bible there are two beginnings—that of the Old Testament and that of the New—so in immunology there are two beginnings: one is *phylogeny*, the other is *ontogeny*.

Phylogeny of the immune response

Phylogeny (*phylo* = race + *geny* = birth) considers the *birth* of the immune system within the *evolutionary* development of the animal *race*. Phylogenists seek to make out a case for the presence of some form of IR as early as the *invertebrates*. Certainly, the invertebrates have their own forms of defence mechanisms—the evidence is in their survival these many millions of years. By stretching the imagination, one may even conjure up some primitive form of immunology in the invertebrates. But we remain sceptical. Nothing in the invertebrate animal looks like immunology to us: Ab is absent and neither specificity nor memory, the hallmarks of the IR, are unequivocally present.

Therefore, we may consider immunology—as we will view it—to begin with the *vertebrates*. *Lymphocytes*, primitive *spleen* and *thymus*, both *humoral* and *cellular* IR, as well as (most definitively) *specificity* and *memory*, are all present in the earliest of vertebrate animals: the *Agnatha* (fish without jaws). Advanced fish add *plasma cells*, but it is not till we come to the *mammals* that *lymph nodes* are clearly identifiable.

Ontogeny of the immune response

Ontogeny (*onto* = existing things) deals with the *development* of the animal from its origin in a fertilized egg to the end product: the *existing* adult animal. The *ability* to mount an IR (termed **immune competence**) similarly develops progressively, but the *maturation stages* in relation to fetal and post-fetal life *vary* between animals: the mouse is born immunologically immature, whereas the lamb is born with most of its immune capacities developed. Also, as shown by investigations in the fetal lamb, *immunological maturation differs*

sequentially in terms of specific antigens, i.e. immune competence to antigen X may be present at, say, day 68 of fetal life, whereas competence to antigen Y may not be developed till day 93. It is during the ontogeny of the IR that self Ags make themselves known to the immune system, thus avoiding development of immune competence (and, later, IR) to self tissues.

THE CELL

Biologically speaking, the primordial function of every living organism is to produce a succeeding generation of its own kind. In Biblical terms, this is embodied in the command to 'go forth and multiply'.

As the identity of an organism lies encoded in its germ plasm—i.e. its genes—the function of the living organism, speaking teleologically, is to pass along its genes to a new generation.

The cell is the basic unit of the living organism. In unicellular organisms, the cell *is* the organism: all functions necessary to maintain the organism are operable in the one cell. So, the function of the unicellular organism becomes simply *to keep itself alive* until it can divide, multiply and, carrying its parcel of duplicated genes with it, become the new generation.

In the *multicellular* organism (apart from mere multicellular colonies), the situation is different. Complexity of structure brings complexities in function—or vice versa. The organism is no longer capable of producing the next generation simply by dividing itself. The mission of procreation resides solely in a particular line of cells: the *germ* cells. The rest of the cells—the *somatic* (*soma* = body) cells—serve solely *to keep the organism alive* until such time as the germ cells can accomplish their procreative mission.

A parallel of this on a social scale is found in the organization of a bee colony. The sole purpose of the colony is—no, not to provide honey for humans!—to insure the survival of the queen bee (the 'germ' bee) so that she can pass on the community's genes to new generations. To this end, the functions of all non-queens (the 'somatic' bees) are directed toward preserving the queen and the hive: constructing and maintaining the hive, gathering nectar, protecting the hive against threats, fertilizing the queen, nourishing and rearing the new generation which comes from the eggs she lays.

Similarly, by the time we get to the higher organisms, different groups of somatic cells take up various functions, the sum total of which provides for the construction, nourishment and protection of the organism until—barring accidents—maturation of its germ cells permits it to pass its genes on to a new generation. In this way we come to have epidermal cells, muscle cells, hepatic cells, renal cells, haematopoietic cells. . . .

And then there are the cells of the immune system. To these cells has been entrusted the defence of the 'organismal realm'. Their prime task is to preserve the organism by warding off attack from without by enemy organisms: bacteria, viruses, worms, etc.—a task for which they are peculiarly adapted.

But, as Gertrude Stein might have said—had she thought along those lines—a cell is a cell is a. . . That is, though cells may differ in form, as dictated by their respective functions, basically they share a common anatomy: a blob of *cytoplasm* in which are embedded a *nucleus* and a variety of *organelles*, the whole enclosed in a *membrane*.

The cells of the immune system are no exception, so an insight to cell anatomy and cell physiology will prove useful for the understanding of otherwise awesome features and activities of immunologically active cells and their products: *surface immunoglobulins, surface markers, major histocompatibility antigens, receptors, rough endoplasmic reticulum, agglutination, rosetting, uptake of radioactive labels*, etc—all formidable terms, yet simple in the context of cell architecture and cell function.

The anatomy of the cell

The nucleus (= kernel) Literally the hereditary 'keys to the kingdom', in that it contains (apart from the mitochondria) all the genetic information gathered within the organism during the eons of its evolution; this information is encoded in the *deoxyribonucleic acid (DNA)* which makes up the chromatin mass of the nucleus.

Chromatin (= coloured material) Packed strands of deoxyribonucleic acid and protein, staining with basic dyes to give the nucleus its characteristic blue colour in stained cells; in the non-dividing cell it is formless, but during mitosis it becomes organized into individual *chromosomes*.

DNA A two-stranded thread, coiled in the form of a double helix; each strand is a chain of nucleotides, each *nucleotide* being comprised of a purine (adenine,

guanine) or pyrimidine (thymine, cytosine) molecule and a molecule of deoxyribose (together comprising a *nucleoside*), plus a molecule of phosphoric acid—all linked together chemically; three adjacent nucleotides make up a *codon,* coding for a triad of complementary nucleotides on a *messenger ribonucleic acid (mRNA),* the mRNA triad in turn coding for a particular amino acid; the sum total of DNA codons carrying the information for *producing* a complete protein is a **gene** (= to produce); with the gene acting as a template, its information is transcribed into a molecule of mRNA; for the convenience of the immunologist, as we shall see, *thymine* is unique to DNA.

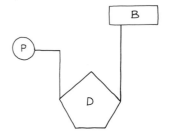

Basic structure of a DNA nucleotide,
composed of : P = phosphate;
                    D = deoxyribose;
                    B = purine or pyrimidine base.

Figure 3.

mRNA A single-stranded nucleic acid in which *uracil* takes the place of thymine and *ribose* replaces deoxyribose; carries the code (*message*) for a single protein from the nucleus to the site of protein synthesis in the cytoplasm.

Chromosome An identifiably-shaped concentration of chromatin, taking the form of two identical clubs (**chromatids**) joined, like Siamese twins, at one point (the **centromere**); as with Siamese twins, the place of joining is variable; so, too, is the size of the chromatids; thus, individual chromosomes can be identified (and given an identifying number) by the length of their chromatids and position of the centromere; since cells carry two of each chromosome—one having come from each parent—they are referred to as **diploid** (= double) cells.

Nucleolus A compact organelle within the nucleus, composed largely of RNA; identified as the seat of production of *ribosomal RNA (rRNA)* for export to the cytoplasm.

Nuclear envelope A membrane-like structure enclosing the nucleus; pierced by **nuclear pores,** which allows

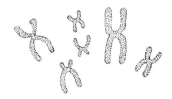

Examples of chromosomes, illustrating the different sizes and different positions of the centromeres.

Figure 4.

traffic of substances between nucleus and cytoplasm.

The cytoplasm (*cyto* = cell + *plasm* = form) A viscid, aqueous solution filling all intracellular space and containing a number of inclusions; rich in proteins, many required for cell maintenance; in addition to the nucleus, other cytoplasmic inclusions are a *cytoskeleton*, which gives form to the cell, and a variety of *organelles* required for cell metabolism and cell function.

The organelles (= little organs):

Cytoskeleton A collection of *microtubules* and *microfilaments* which radiate throughout the cell; as well as determining cell form, they also determine cell movement in motile cells.

Centriole A paired structure, each of the pair consisting of a *bundle of parallel microtubules*, sited near the *centre* of the resting (i.e. non-dividing) cell.

Endoplasmic reticulum A *network* (*rete* = net) of sheet- or tube-like structures lying within (= *endo*) and running through the cytoplasm; seen in *two forms:* **smooth** and **rough**; the rough appearance of the latter is tied up with its function in the synthesis of protein and is due to its surface being studded with knobby *ribosomes*, the seats of protein synthesis; the more actively a cell is synthesizing protein, the more prominent its rough endoplasmic reticulum.

Ribosome A body composed of protein and of RNA; acts as a point of attachment for mRNA coming from the nucleus; one mRNA molecule usually attaches to several ribosomes to form a **polysome** (*poly* = several); here the mRNA assumes its role as *template* for the synthesis of protein, the requisite amino acids being brought to it by *specific transfer RNA (tRNA)*.

tRNA A small RNA molecule carrying two specific codes: one for a particular amino acid, the other to recognize the proper triad on the mRNA at which to deposit that amino acid; hence, **transfer RNA.**

Golgi apparatus A multifunctional collection of tubules and sacs, forming a dish-shaped structure lying to one side of the nucleus; among its functions is that of *glycosylation of proteins*, important, for example, in the attachment of the carbohydrate groups to immuno-

globulin heavy chains; also, lytic proteins (enzymes) are here packaged as **lysosomes**; while proteins for export (e.g. immunoglobulins in plasma cells) are packaged into **secretory vacuoles**.

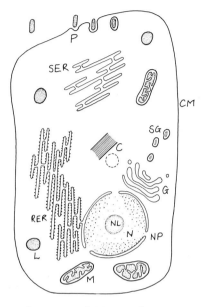

Schematic diagram of a cell.

C = pair of centrioles, with long axes at right angles to each other;	P = steps in phagocyte formation;
CM = cell membrane;	RER = rough endoplasmic reticulum;
G = golgi apparatus;	SER = smooth endoplasmic reticulum;
L = lysosome;	SG = secretory granules;
N = nucleus;	cytoskeleton not shown.
NL = nucleolus;	
NP = nuclear pore;	

Figure 5.

Lysosome (= dissolving body) Primarily involved in intracellular digestion of phagocytosed or pinocytosed matter; latter is engulfed by protoplasmic extensions of the cell and taken into the cell in a vacuole—a **phagosome** (= eating body)—formed by fusion of the cell membrane around it; lysosome and phagosome fuse, exposing the phagocytosed matter to enzymatic lysis; some cells—particularly neutrophils—when activated will expel the lysosomal enzymes into surrounding tissue, causing tissue damage.

Secretory vacuole Carries export proteins to the cell membrane, fuses with the membrane and expels its contents from the cell for use elsewhere in the body.

Mitochondria Generally oval-shaped bodies with internal partitions extending from the inner wall; may in the distant past have been independent organisms which settled in a cell and became part of the cell machinery;

certainly, they still carry independent DNA for synthesis of their own proteins and divide into daughter mitochondria during cell mitosis; in the cell they function as *power-generators*, oxidizing sugars to generate energy (in the form of energy-rich *adenosine triphosphate: ATP*) required by the rest of the cell.

Granules Organized aggregates of active components, found in different numbers and sizes in different cells; of particular interest to the immunologist are the prominent granules of mast cells, basophils and neutrophils.

Cell membrane A double layer of closely packed *phospholipid* molecules, each shaped like a two-tailed tadpole: a **hydrophilic** (*hydro* = water + *philic* = loving) head with two **hydrophobic** (= water hating) tails; the

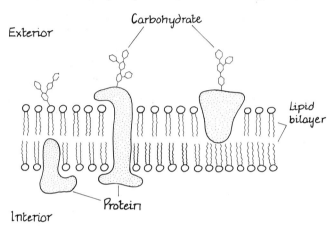

A cross-sectional view of a cell membrane; the constituents are not rigidly fixed but can move freely in the plane of the membrane.

Figure 6.

membrane is formed by two sheets of lipid molecules lying tail to tail, with the hydrophilic heads forming the inner and outer surfaces of the cell membrane; associated with the lipid membrane are a variety of *proteins, many embedded in the membrane* like currants in a bun; some of the embedded proteins are exposed at the outer surface of the membrane, in which situation they are *accessible antigens* to which antibodies can be raised in other animals; such antisera can then be used to characterize the nature of the proteins and to identify the cells with which they are associated; viewed in this light, such things as histocompatibility antigens, surface markers, receptors are reduced to a common denominator (regardless of the complexity of the nomenclature accorded them by the immunologist) and shed the awesomeness of the esoteric; **histocompatibility antigens** simply become membrane proteins that happen to be

coded for by the histocompatibility region genes in the chromosome; **surface markers** are simply membrane proteins which can be associated with a particular type, set or sub-set of cells; **receptors** are simply membrane proteins which can latch onto another molecule; thus, an **immunoglobulin receptor** is simply a membrane protein which can latch on to an immunoglobulin heavy chain; *it is all simplicity itself*.

The activities of the cell

Mitosis

This is the **cell transformation** of immunological jargon. But 'mitosis' or 'cell transformation', cell division by any other name is still *cell division*.

The division of cells to replenish lost cells, or to increase the numbers of existing cells, is fundamental to life itself. Most nucleated cells are capable of mitosis. Those which are not—e.g. plasma cells—are designated terminal, or *end cells*: they are the *end* of the line.

When a cell divides, it must furnish its daughter cells with a sufficiency of cytoplasm, plus its entire repertoire of genetic information. To do so, it must *manufacture more cytoplasmic protein* and *duplicate its chromatin*. These are the major phenomena associated with mitosis. Though certainly not designed for that purpose, these phenomena prove exceedingly useful to the immunologist.

Mitosis begins with an increase of rough endoplasmic reticulum, needed for the synthesis of the additional protein required. This *increases the size of the cell* and *loads the cytoplasm with ribosomal RNA*. This is what the immunologist calls the **blast cell**. Also, because it is large and the RNA takes the red stain of pyronin, it is referred to as the **large pyroninophilic cell**. The immunologist looks for this cell as a sign of transformation.

The centrioles are duplicated, each pair then migrating to opposite poles of the cell. Between them is stretched a spindle-shaped scaffolding of microtubules: the **mitotic spindle**.

Meanwhile, the chromatin is organizing itself into chromosomes. These attach themselves to the tubules in the middle of the spindle. The centromeres of each chromosome split, allowing the two chromatids to separate (= **chromatid separation**), each being drawn to opposite ends of the spindle. Here they replicate to restore the original diploid set of chromosomes.

Now the cell can divide. It does so by pinching in its cytoplasm in the middle, following up with fusion of the cell membrane to seal off the two daughter cells.

The replication of the chromosomes in mitosis affords the immunologist a useful tool for the study of factors associated with cell transformation. Since new strands of DNA synthesized in the process will incorporate within their structure available precursor molecules, a radioactively labelled precursor can be used for the quantitation of transformation in particular immunological situations. Commonly, the radioactive tritiated form of the thymidine nucleoside (containing the conveniently DNA-specific thymine) is introduced into the system under study. After a suitable incubation period, measuring the radioactivity of the washed cells determines the degree of incorporation of tritiated thymidine, which in turn is an index to the cell transformation which has taken place.

Meiosis

When a somatic cell undergoes mitosis it produces two diploid daughter cells. This is as it should be, as cell identity and function must be preserved.

But, obviously, such diploid duplication cannot be tolerated in reproduction. If **gametes** (= the fertilizing cells) had diploid numbers of chromosomes, when they came together in fertilization they would produce a tetraploid individual, which would, in turn, give rise to an octaploid organism, and so on ad infinitum. Where would it ever end?

To avoid this impossible situation, Nature has introduced the process of **meiosis** (= lessening) in the production of gametes from germ cells. During meiosis the chromosome pairs are separated into two separate sets, each set containing one chromosome from each pair. When the cell divides, one set goes to each of the two gametes produced. In this way gametes have a lesser—i.e. **haploid** (= single)—number of chromosomes. The diploid number is restored in the next generation by fusion of the nuclei of the two gametes, which come together when fertilization occurs.

As separation of the chromosome pairs in meiosis is purely random, siblings will differ from each other in the genetic information they inherit from each parent. In immunological terms, they may be different in terms of histocompatibility, and so not tolerate each others tissues, and their immune systems may behave differently to antigenic stimuli.

To eliminate such troublesome variables from his experimental animals, the immunologist has created **inbred strains** of animals. By repeated selective offspring-parent and brother-sister matings over many generations, the genetic variability is reduced and finally eliminated to produce a **syngeneic** (= created alike) strain of animal, in which all individuals are genetically alike. In man, **identical twins**—which arise by splitting of the same pair of fused gametes—are syngeneic and will perfectly tolerate each others tissues: an ideal situation when an organ transplant is required.

Gene expression

Within an organism, every somatic cell has exactly the same packet of genes—which it inherited from its progenitor gametes—as every other cell. Why, then—and how—do they differ in appearance and function?

The answer lies in **gene expression**.

Only in the unicellular organism are all functional genes expressed in one cell. In the multicellular animal, there is a built-in on/off mechanism, which allows in any one cell the *expression* (i.e. activation) only of those genes required for the maintenance of the cell and the performance of its specific function. The other genes are **repressed**: they lie dormant and inactive. For example, in a thyroid cell are expressed those genes coding for thyroglobulin; in the Langerhans cells of the pancreas, those genes coding for insulin; in the erythroblast, those genes coding for the haemoglobin required by the erythrocyte; and so on.

Similarly, the nature of the proteins in the membrane of a cell is determined by which of the various genes coding for membrane proteins are expressed. This can be independent of other gene expression. Thus, two cells which have identical histocompatibility Ags and look morphologically similar, may, because of differences in gene expression of their membrane proteins, manifest certain unique Ags in their cell membranes, which sets one apart from the other on serological examination. Thus, it is simply such gene expression which accounts for the differences in surface markers between B lymphocytes and T lymphocytes, as well as between subsets of each.

Mutation

The very existence of the inexhaustible number of plant and animal species is silent testimony to the phenomenon of **mutation** (= change), as mutation is the origin of species variability.

If transmissible change is to be introduced into living systems, it must come about by change in the genetic code in its passage from generation to generation. Such change seems to arise spontaneously and at random, and is probably triggered off by factors in the environment: e.g. chemicals or radiations which alter the nucleotide composition of the DNA. It may be the aggregation of such mutant genes by selective breeding which enables the immunologist to produce nude mice and obese chickens.

Though mutation would appear to be a phenomenon related to reproduction, there is a school of thought which holds that mutations which influence somatic events can also take place in the course of the ontogeny of the individual. This leads to the split between those holding a genetic view and others holding a somatic view of antibody diversity. While the geneticists hold that all the information required for the production of the individual's entire repertoire of immunoglobulins is passed along by the germ cells (= the **germ line theory**), the somaticists insist this is only partially true and that the genetic information must be supplemented by somatic mutation (= the **somatic mutation theory**). Both produce evidence to support their own viewpoints.

THE GENE

The **gene** (*gen* = to produce), a strand of deoxyribo-nucleic acid (**DNA**) a few hundred or thousand purine/pyrimidine bases long, is the sole *raison d'être* of the cell: it is the basis of heredity. It carries the information needed to produce a single protein, which will influence a single hereditary characteristic.

Two genes, each lying in one of a matching pair of chromosomes, control one particular characteristic. They are called **alleles** (= of one another); the *place* each occupies is called a **locus** (pl. **loci**). If both alleles at one locus code for the *same* form of the characteristic (e.g. blue eyes), they are said to be **homozygous** (*homo* = same); if *different* (i.e. one blue, one brown), they are said to be **heterozygous** (*hetero* = other). The *gene combination* at a locus determines the **genotype** of an individual; the *actual expression* of the gene characteristic determines the **phenotype** (*pheno* = to show). If in a heterozygous situation *both genes* at a locus are expressed, they are said to be **co-dominant**; if only *one* is expressed, it is a *dominant* gene, while the *non-expressed* gene is a *recessive* gene. The *suppression* of expression of one gene by its allele is called **allelic exclusion**. If both alleles are recessive, then the characteristic will be expressed. Though individually each gene represents an infinitesimal fragment of a chromosome, collectively the genes produce the individual and dictate the nature of its individuality.

Fundamental to the role of the gene is its primordial function of reproducing itself for transmission to the next generation. In fact, a new science springing up under the name of sociobiology, claims that all of life,

reproduction and evolution is nothing more than the expression of the gene's ruthless struggle for self-perpetuation.

It is thus surprising that the gene is a johnny-come-lately on the immunological scene. Though its influence was noted as early as 1900 in relation to the inheritance of blood groups, it is only since the 1950s that its fundamental role in the IR has been unfolded.

The work of Medawar and his colleagues on the rejection of tissue grafts between members of the same species brought the realization that even individuals within a species differ from each other in terms of the *immunological uniqueness* of the Ags sitting on their cell membranes. Startling as this revelation was at the time, it could have been anticipated, considering all the other differences there are between members of a species: eye colour, hair colour and texture, height, build, etc.

The following words are commonly associated with genetic relationship between individuals.

Syngeneic *Complete genetic identity* between individuals of the same species, such as between *identical* twins and between individuals of an *in-bred strain* of animals.

Identical twin Twins arising from the *same* fertilized egg.

In-bred Parent-offspring and brother-sister mating over many generations to produce a strain of animals in which all individuals manifest *genetic identity*: one member will accept any tissue from any other member of the same strain, while rejecting tissues from animals of different strains.

Congenic In-bred strains differing from each other only in one inherited character.

Allogeneic Genetically determined differences between members of the same species.

Xenogeneic Completely foreign, as between different species of animals.

Histocompatibility Ags (HAs) Genetically defined Ags present on the surface of all body cells except the RBC; first recognized for their nuisance role in the rejection of tissue transplants (hence, also, **transplantation Ags**), bringing the concept that tissues contain Ags which must be *compatible* (identical) between donor and recipient for graft acceptance; thus, fundamental to the recognition of **self** and **non-self** (i.e. that which is antigenically **identical** or **non-identical** with an individual's own HAs). The individuality of HAs is under control of a closely linked set (= complex) of genes occupying a small portion of a single chromosome (no. 6 in man; no. 17 in mouse) and collectively known as the **major histocompatibility complex,** or **MHC**; also termed the **HLA (human leucocyte antigen) region** in *man* and the **H-2**

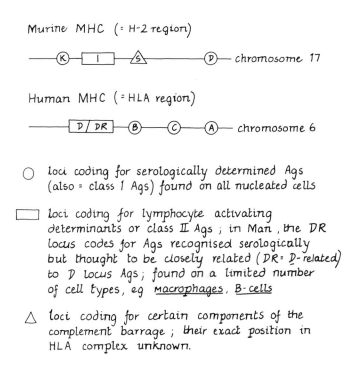

Murine MHC (= H-2 region)

Human MHC (= HLA region)

○ loci coding for serologically determined Ags (also = class 1 Ags) found on all nucleated cells

☐ loci coding for lymphocyte activating determinants or class II Ags ; in Man , the DR locus codes for Ags recognised serologically but thought to be closely related (DR = D-related) to D locus Ags ; found on a limited number of cell types, eg macrophages , B-cells

△ loci coding for certain components of the complement barrage ; their exact position in HLA complex unknown.

Figure 7. Simplified major histocompatibility complexes.

region in the *mouse* (Figure 7). The HAs coded by the MHC genes include some which can be identified by *antisera* prepared by immunization of unrelated strains of animals, or spontaneously produced in pregnant mothers carrying embryos with unrelated paternal HAs (= **serologically determined; SD**). Other HAs only become evident in *mixed lymphocyte culture* (hence, **MLC Ags**), in which situation the contact between two MHC-incompatible lymphocytes in the culture causes them to *react* by enlarging and dividing (hence, *mixed lymphocyte reaction:* **MLR**)—further, as *lymphocyte activation* is involved in the *determination* of these MHC Ags, they are also referred to as **LADs** (= *lymphocyte activating determinants*).

HAEMATOPOIETIC TISSUE

Returning to our Bible analogy in the context of ontogeny, in the beginning there are the *haematopoietic tissues*, which 'beget' the cells of the blood and lymphoid organs, from which is 'begat' immunology itself.

Haematopoietic tissues are those tissues containing the **stem cells**, which are the producers (*poietic* = making) of the *formed elements* of the blood (*haemato*); earliest location is in the embryo yolk sac, moving on to the fetal liver and finally to the bone marrow, the latter being the sole site in the normal adult.

BLOOD

Formed elements Those parts of the blood which are solid *(formed)* in nature — i.e. the **blood cells**:

Erythrocyte The red (= *erythro*) blood cell (= *cyte*): **RBC**; carries in its cell membrane many genetically defined Ags (= **blood group substances**) which determine **blood groups: A, B, O; Rh+, Rh−**; *et al.*

Leucocytes The white (= *leuco*) blood cells: **WBC**; these are *wandering* cells, leaving the blood stream to patrol the tissues, or making a massive invasion of a particular area in response to chemical call to action: **chemotaxis** (= *chemical attraction*); types of leucocytes are:

Mononuclear cells A collective term for the lymphocytes and monocytes, in which the nucleus is discretely single (= *mono*).

Lymphocyte Small cell with discrete, compact, round nucleus and very little cytoplasm; *circulates* in blood and lymphatic vessels, *patrols* through tissues and is *mobilised* in the secondary lymphoid organs. Though indistinguishable in appearance, lymphocytes come in several distinct functional types (= **sets**)— the T-cells and B-cells, and their *sub-sets*—which together form the core of the immunological system. They contain genetically defined cell membrane Ags, some of which (HLA, H-2) are associated with the *histocompatibility* (or tissue) uniqueness of the individuals within a species; others are characteristic for the lymphocyte set or subset on which they occur; yet others are *recognition receptors* for Ag epitopes, each cell containing receptors for *one* specific epitope. Originally in a quiescent form, a lymphocyte becomes **activated** (= *primed*) on contact with Ag carrying an epitope for which it has a recognition receptor.

Null cell Cell with the morphological characteristics of lymphocytes, but lacking the surface markers and functional properties of T- or B-cells; therefore, they form a third set of peripheral blood lymphocytes.

Natural killer cell (NK cell) More readily described by functional than by structural properties; NK cells express *natural cytotoxic activity in the non-immune individual* against certain target cells, such as tumour and virally-infected cells. This activity appears to be confined to cells with receptors for IgG, which are known as *large granular lymphocytes*, and it is enhanced by *interferon*. The precise role of these cells in IR and IRC is not known, but they have been implicated in tumour surveillance, defence against viral infections, and transplant rejection.

Monocyte Nucleus generally indented and surrounded by clear cytoplasm; cytoplasm is characterized by abundance of enzyme-containing *lysosomes*; cell is large (= *macro*) and phagocytic (*phago* = eat), so also called a **macrophage** (designated **Mφ**); **phagocytosis** involves adhesion to and engulfment of insoluble particles; soluble substances are engulfed within small liquid droplets: **pinocytosis** (*pino* = drink). In this way it takes in both insoluble and soluble Ags for *processing* prior to *presentation* to the lymphoid system; has membrane surface receptors for *Fc* of IgG Ab and *C3b* from complement.

Granulocytes Three types of leucocytes characterized by *granules* in the cytoplasm. *Nucleus* is variably segmented—i.e. comes in many forms (= **polymorphic**)—so also collectively known as the **polymorphonuclear cells,** or **polymorphs;** comprised of:

Eosinophil Cell with large granules staining bright *red* with *eosin* (+*phil* = love). Can take in Ag-Ab complexes; rushes to site of *anaphylactic reaction*; prominent in *worm infestation* and has been shown to damage some worms in presence of *IgE* Ab, but role not fully understood.

Basophil The large granules stain deep *blue* with *basic* dyes. Granules are packed with pharmacologically active chemicals and packaged in **perigranular** (*peri* = all around) **membrane**; these chemicals, generally referred to as **mediators** (i.e. they *mediate* certain physiological activities of tissues and cells), are released in *anaphylactic* and *complement-fixing* situations. Membrane has receptors for *Fc* region of *IgE*.

Neutrophil Contains smaller, weakly pink-staining (hence, *neutral*) granules; *phagocytic* in function, but smaller (*micro*) than the Mφ, so also known as **microphage**. Granules contain enzymes which kill and digest phagocytosed microorganisms and damaged cells; rushes to site of *complement activation* and inflammation. Primary role is scavenging, in the course of which it kills itself, so releasing its enzymes and causing tissue damage; also known as **'suicide cell'**.

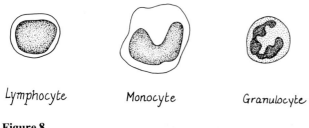

Lymphocyte   Monocyte   Granulocyte

Figure 8.

K cell Leucocyte bearing receptors for Ab Fc and so capable of participating in the *killing* of Ab coated cells (= **Ab-dependent cell-mediated cytotoxicity — ADCC**).

Thrombocyte More commonly called **platelet**; minute, nonnucleated, formed element involved primarily in blood clotting mechanism (*thrombus* = clot); rich in HAs and some anaphylactic mediators.

Humoral elements Cell products which make up the *soluble* substances contained in the fluid portion of the blood, the **blood plasma**, separated from *unclotted* blood by spinning off the cells; some are proteins associated with IR and IRC: *immunoglobulins, complement components, kininogen*.

Immunoglobulins (Ig) A *family* of blood glycoproteins sharing in common a *globular* structure and identified with the *immunologically* active Abs; perhaps best differentiated thus: an Ab is an Ig for which a specific Ag-binding function has been established; on **electrophoretic** (*phoros* = carry, i.e. carried by an electric current) separation of serum proteins, the Igs move slowly, lagging behind in the *gamma* region, so also termed **gammaglobulins**; have numerous roles in immune defence and IRC.

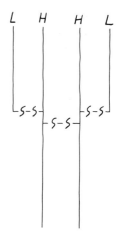

Figure 9. Basic 4-chain structure of an Ig molecule, where L = light chain and H = heavy chain.

Structure In its basic form an Ig molecule has a 4-chain structure (Figure 9), made up of one pair of identical **heavy (H)** chains of mol. wt ca. 50,000–65,000 and one pair of identical **light (L)** chains of mol. wt ca. 25,000; the two H chains are bound to each other by **interchain** (*inter* = between) **disulfide bridges** (-S-S-); one L chain is bound to each H chain by an interchain -S-S-; knowledge of the 4-chain structure of the Ig molecule is based on chemical splitting of the -S-S- and isolation and identification of the individual chains.

(In thinking about Igs, I have been struck by the parallels between Igs and human fingers (Fi).

Therefore, I have drawn a number of analogies between them. G.F.)

Immunoglobulin classes *Five* distinct Ig classes have been identified; they have been named: *IgM, IgG, IgD, IgA, IgE*; they are recognizably different from each other, as are the fingers of the hand, which could be similarly put into classes; *FiT* (thumb), *FiI* (index), *FiM* (middle), *FiR* (ring), *FiL* (little); the different Ig classes have different biological properties and different heavy chains; but they all share the same two types of light chain.

Immunoglobulin sub-classes Within the *IgG* and *IgA* classes further differences in structure and biological activities define *sub-classes*; four sub-classes of IgG in *man* have been named IgG1, IgG2, IgG3, IgG4; IgA sub-classes are: IgA1 and IgA2; they occur together in all individuals; in the finger analogy, each class has two sub-classes, left (1) and right (2) FiT1, FiT2, FiI1, FiI2.

. . . .

Heavy chains (H chains) *Polypeptide* chains of *five* different varieties—μ, γ, δ, α, ϵ—respectively corresponding to the Ig classes: IgM, IgG, IgD, IgA, IgE; H chains are made up of ca. 440 (γ, α) or ca. 550 (μ, δ, ϵ) *amino acids (a.a.)*, plus attached carbohydrate groups. Chain identities are established by production of and reaction with specific antisera: e.g. animal immunized with α-chain will produce anti-α antiserum, which will combine with α-chains. The biological properties characteristic for each Ig class are determined by the polypeptide structure of its H chain.

a.a. sequencing Chemical methods for determining the *sequence of* **a.a.**s in the H chain show there is a *free amino ($-NH_2$)* group at one end (**N-terminal end**) and a free *carboxyl ($-COOH$)* group at the other end (**C-terminal end**). *Numbering* of the a.a.s along the chain starts from the N-terminal end; a.a. sequencing further shows the chain can be divided into 4 (α, γ) or 5 (μ, δ, ϵ) sub-units of ca. 110 a.a.s, each characterized by the presence of a ca. 60 a.a. loop closed by an **intrachain** (*intra* = within) -S-S-. Each such sub-unit is termed a **domain** (loosely, like the sections of the fingers).

Starting from the N-terminal end, the a.a. sequence forming the region of the first domain of the H chain *varies* markedly—not only from the a.a. sequence in subsequent domains on the same chain, but also from the N-terminal domain of other H chains—hence: **variable heavy region, variable heavy domain (V_H—** diagramatically symbolized: ⋀⋀⋀⋀). The variability is produced by the possibility of two or more alternate a.a.s occupying the same position in the polypeptide chain—e.g. a choice between leucine, glycine and alanine at position 24, between valine and tyrosine at pos. 45, etc.

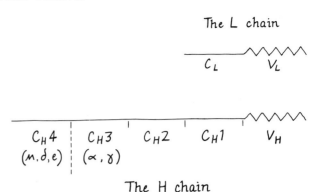

Figure 10.

Within the V_H are found four separate groups of ca. 6–10 a.a.s, these groups being *even more variable* than the rest of the domain (i.e. the choice between alternative a.a.s is even greater than at other V domain positions); hence: **hypervariable** (*hyper* = greater) **regions** or '*hot spots*'; these regions are of particular significance for the *Ag-binding specificity* of the Ig molecule.

Those parts of V_H and V_L not in the hypervariable regions, but providing support for them, are known as the **framework** regions; variability in these regions can (also) be responsible for *isotypy* and *idiotypy*.

By contrast, not only is the sequence in the a.a. region ca. 110–440/550 relatively *constant* (**constant region**, diagramatically: —————), but also each of the 3 or 4 domains within the constant region is remarkably similar to the other domains in the constant region and to comparable domains on other chains; hence: **constant domains**, designated in order following V_H: C_H1, C_H2, C_H3, plus, in μ, δ, and ϵ chains, C_H4—i.e. *first constant heavy domain*, etc.

Between C_H1 and C_H2 the H chain is very flexible by virtue of a sequence of *proline* a.a.s; as the chain can *bend* and *unbend* at this point, it is termed the **hinge region** (Figure 11).

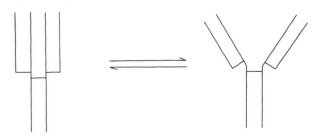

Figure 11. Flexibility in the hinge region.

Light chains (L chains) Polypeptide chains of ca. 220 a.a.s, made up of *one variable* L domain (V_L) and *one constant* light domain (C_L); two types of light chain exist, termed **kappa** (κ) and **lambda** (λ), which can be identified by their specific reaction with *anti-κ* and *anti-λ* respectively. Both κ and λ chains occur in *all* Ig classes, but on any one Ig molecule *both* light chains are of the *same* type (e.g. $\kappa_2\alpha_2$ or $\lambda_2\alpha_2$). V_L contains 3 *hypervariable* regions, the combination of which with the 4 hypervariable regions of the H chain produces the Ab **paratope**: i.e. the particular structure on the *Fab* which is complementary to and makes a close fit for the epitope on the Ag, thus giving the Ab its specificity in Ag recognition and combination. It is apparent that, with 6–10 very variable a.a. positions in each of the 7 hypervariable regions making up the paratope, the combination can produce specificities for thousands of different epitopes.

Immunoglobulin fragments Igs can also be *split by proteolytic enzymes; papain* splits the H chain of IgG in a manner which produces *two identical fragments* which can still bind with Ag: **Fab** (*= fragment antigen-binding*), each made up of an intact L chain linked via the L-H -S-S- to the N-terminal portion of the H chain. The two C-terminal portions of H chains are still linked to each other by the H-H -S-S- to form a *third fragment* which crystallizes from solution: **Fc** (*= fragment crystallizable*).

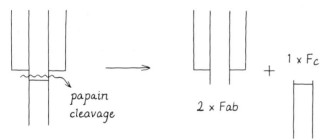

Figure 12.

Since the Fab still carries one complete paratope, it retains the *immunological* property of binding with Ag; but since it is **monovalent** (*mono* = one + *valent* = power) it is *incapable of cross-linking* Ags to produce *precipitation* or *agglutination*.

Certain *biological* properties of the Igs are the function of the Fc fragment: transport through the placenta (IgG), fixing of complement (IgG, IgM), attachment to mast cells and basophils (IgE), attachment to WBCs.

If the enzyme *pepsin* is used to split IgG, the -S-S- between the two H chains remains with the Fab fragments, linking them together to yield *one* **F(ab′)$_2$** fragment; the remaining portions of the H chains are no longer joined together, so no intact Fc is obtained.

Since F(ab′)$_2$ is *divalent* (*di* = two), it can link together Ags to precipitate or agglutinate them.

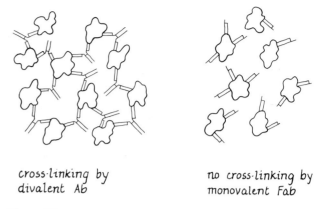

cross-linking by
divalent Ab

no cross-linking by
monovalent Fab

Figure 13.

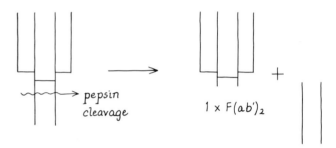

pepsin
cleavage

1 × F(ab′)$_2$

Figure 14.

Genetic variants The a.a. sequence of the chains of an Ig molecule is determined by the genes inherited by the individual from its parents; as in all other inherited characteristics (e.g. fingers), time, mutation and evolution have introduced some transmissible variations in DNA structure which are translated into variations in the a.a. sequence structure of the Ig chains: i.e. *substitution* of one a.a. for another at a particular point in the chain. These variations, termed **genetic markers**, are detectable by interaction of the Ig variants with specific antisera raised against them; such studies have shown that Ig variants are of three principal types.

Isotypes Variants found side by side in the *same (iso) individual*: i.e. they are all normally inherited by *all members* of a species (e.g. the five different fingers on the human hand). In this sense the 5 different *classes* of Ig are isotypes, since we all normally inherit them just as we do our 5 different Fi; within the classes IgG and IgA are found further a.a. sequence variations giving rise to *sub-classes*, which occur in all individuals, so also qualifying as isotypes. (Here we can recognize our Fi1s and Fi2s as being isotypes, as we all have them.) The a.a. sequence variations between Ig classes and sub-classes are found in the C_H regions. The κ and λ *types of* L chains are also isotypes, as are two *subtypes* (Oz$^+$ and Oz$^-$) of the λ chain; additionally, certain a.a. sequence variations in the framework regions of V_L and V_H give rise to further isotypes, which are termed *sub-groups*. Functional differences have been established for Ig classes and sub-classes, but not for the other isotypes.

Allotypes A genetic *either/or* situation. Individuals of the same species may differ (such as in the overall length and shape of fingers: *either* long *or* short, *either* thick *or* thin). Genetic information controlling the a.a. sequence of Ig chains permits *either* one *or* another (= *allo*) a.a. to occupy a particular position in the Ig chain; each a.a. influences its own shape of epitope at that particular part of the chain, each epitope representing a different allotype. However, since the alleles coding for these allotypes are co-dominant, two allotypes will co-exist in the heterozygous individual; **Gm** (*m* for *marker*) allotypes and **Am** allotypes are determined by a.a. variations on the γ and α H chains respectively, and so are found only in IgG and IgA; but **Km** are found on all κ chains and thus in all Ig classes. No functional role has been established for the allotypes, which are identified solely by their ability to induce and react with *anti-allotype* sera.

Idiotypes The simple fact of the great variability in a.a. sequence in the hypervariable region of the H and L chains (and, to a lesser extent, in the framework regions) injects a third type of variability in Ig molecules: that related to *Ag-binding specificity*; a perfect analogy for the idiotype is the fingerprint, in which the great number of potential ridge shape variations insures a combination which is unique for any one fingerprint. Similarly in the Ig *paratopes*, the great number of potential a.a. variations possible in the V_H and V_L hypervariable region insures a combination which is unique for any one Ab; idiotypes are identified by use of *anti-idiotype antisera*. Obviously, the role of the Ig idiotype is to recognize and react with one specific epitope, but near-recognition (i.e. reasonable, though not perfect, fit) enables it to bind with closely similar epitopes, producing the phenomenon of **cross-reaction**.

Complement (C) A set of eleven blood proteins, grouped as nine *components* of the *classical pathway*; there is also an *alternate* pathway which involves certain accessory proteins designated as *factors*. Both of these pathways consist of a chain reaction leading to *inflammation* and which may terminate in *cell death* and *cell lysis*—a process no doubt designed to destroy infective microbial cells, but which not infrequently perversely damages the body's own cells. The components of *C*, in their order of interaction in the classical pathway are labelled C1q, r, s, C4, C2, C3, C5, C6, C7, C8, C9. Since the reaction passes from one component to the next in cascade fashion, it is commonly termed the **complement cascade**; but since this term fails to depict the barrage of biologically active compounds generated in the course of the reaction, we propose the term **complement barrage**.

C3 may be considered the **keystone** (= a part on which other things depend) of the C system. It is the most abundant component and is the focus of the two pathways which, though arising independently in different manner, after activating C3 by splitting it into C3a and C3b, converge into a **common pathway**.

Classical pathway So-called because of its historical priority, and initiated by the combination of the paratopes of IgG or IgM with Ag epitopes to form an **immune complex**. The combination allows C1q (together with C1r and C1s, which come along with it as the C1 complex) to *fix* to the Ab Fc, either because of *high density* of Fc in the complex or as a result of a *structural change* in Fc on binding Ag—i.e. **complement fixation**; the fixed C1 now becomes an enzyme (**C1 esterase**) which splits C4 and then C2 into fragments labelled C4a, C4b, C2a, C2b. In the presence of a cell, the C4b and C2a bind next to each other on the cell membrane to form a new enzyme complex, represented by $\overline{C42}$ (the bar indicates the activated form). $\overline{C42}$ now splits C3 to *convert* it to C3a and C3b (which is why $\overline{C42}$ is also known as **C3 convertase**). C3a has two important activities: it *attracts neutrophils* into the area (**chemotaxis**) (though this is not universally accepted) and produces local inflammation by *degranulating mast cells* (and hence is called an **anaphylotoxin**—i.e. a poison producing an anaphylactic reaction). The C3b, by contrast, binds to cell membrane and complexes with $\overline{C42}$ to form $\overline{C423b}$; here ends the classical pathway.

Alternate (alternative) pathway So called because of its later discovery as an *alternate (alternative)* to the classical pathway; again the objective is the activation of C3, but this time the process is begun by certain *exogenous* compounds: bacterial *endotoxin*, bacterial *polysaccharide*, and yeast wall *zymosan*. *Aggregated IgA* may also activate the alternate pathway. These exogenous compounds act in conjunction with a number of *endogenous* plasma proteins (= **factors**) to enhance the cleavage of C3, the central reaction of the C barrage. Unlike the classical pathway, the alternate pathway is active at low levels in normal serum ('**tick over**') and activation involves simply pushing the system along faster; C3b (some of which is always kicking about) binds with **factor B** and becomes susceptible to cleavage by activated **factor D** ($\overline{D}$). This produces C3bBb (and a fragment Ba) which acts as a **C3 convertase** in a manner analogous to $\overline{C42}$. This C3 convertase, stabilized by

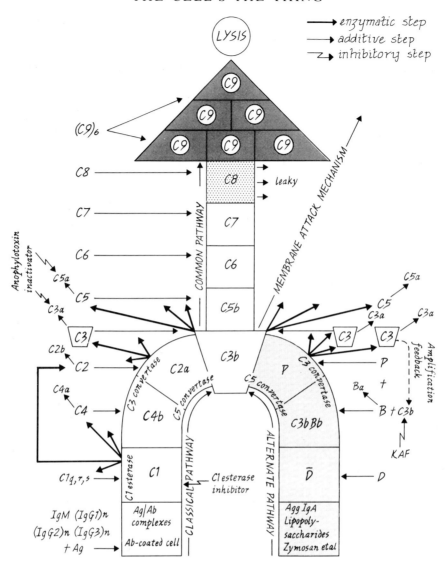

Figure 15.

properdin (**P**), splits C3 into C3a and C3b; the newly generated C3b can in turn combine with factor B to create more C3bBb, which splits more C3, and so on; this is the **alternate pathway loop**, which serves as a **positive feedback amplification mechanism** to augment the C barrage. In normal serum, uncontrolled activation and complete consumption of the body's C3 is prevented by a **C3b inactivator, KAF**. 'Activators' of the alternate pathway shift the balance from this inactivation of C3b via KAF to activation via combination with factor B; some 'activators' stabilize C3bBb itself.

C3b inactivator In the presence of a cofactor, β1H, this converts the active C3b into an inactive form, which is then readily split by trypsin-like enzymes into the fragments C3c and C3d. The inactive form of C3b was long ago observed to bind to bovine konglutinin (German spelling), and C3b inactivator is thus known historically as **konglutinin activating factor (KAF)**; KAF keeps the C3b within bounds and prevents the total destruction of C3. A compound found in cobra venom (**cobra venom factor**, or **cvf**) can combine with B to form CcvfBb, which is a *C3 convertase*. Since cvf is *not* inactivated by KAF, when injected into an animal it creates a self-perpetuating C3 activation loop which soon destroys all the animal's C3; cvf is used experimentally to produce a C-free animal.

Common pathway Having converged in C3b, the classical and alternate pathways now combine to follow a *common course* with a number of key objectives, all with clearly discernible teleological functions in terms of countering infection: to *prepare* the infecting organisms for *phagocytosis* (= **opsonization**: to prepare as food), to call the phagocytes to the site of infection (**chemotaxis**), to allow circulating Ab to escape the confines of the blood vessels and enter the infected tissues (**increased capillary permeability**), and to kill the invading microbial cells directly by *punching holes* in their membranes (**lysis**). Such teleological interpretation of the functions of the C system has adequate corroboration in the observation that persons with hereditary *deficiencies* of one of the C components generally suffer *recurrent*, and sometimes life-threatening, *infections*.

$\overline{C3bBb}$ and $\overline{C423b}$ are also **convertases** for C5, splitting it into C5a, which is chemotactic and anaphylactic, and C5b; the C5b quickly complexes with C6 and C7 to form $\overline{C567}$, which seeks out a cell membrane to sit on. Ideally this is the membrane of an infecting microorganism, but not uncommonly a handy 'innocent bystander' cell serves the purpose (leading, ultimately, to **bystander lysis**). C8 now comes along to join $\overline{C567}$ on the cell membrane, at which stage discrete holes are punched in the membrane and the cell becomes *leaky* and the cytoplasm begins to ooze out. To speed up the process, up to six C9s are attached and act as a *catalyst*, producing a cataclysmic spillage of the cell contents (= **lysis**). Together, the C5 to C9 steps are commonly known as the **membrane attack mechanism**.

The complement barrage The 'big guns' of the C barrage are $\overline{C1}$ and $\overline{C42}$; being an *enzyme*, one unit of C1 can *amplify* the attack by producing many units of $\overline{C42}$. As the latter is also an enzyme, it further amplifies the attack by creating many units of C3b (at which point the *positive feedback amplification loop* can come into play), and then C5b; C8 completes the amplification process (the barrage) by binding up to 6 units of C9.

The teleological functions served by the C barrage are carried out by the molecular fragments and complexes thrown up in the process: *opsonization* — C4b, C3b; *chemotaxis* — C3a, C5a, C567; *increased capillary permeability* — C3a, C5a; *lysis* — C8, C9.

Control mechanisms Since uncontrolled C activation would result in much tissue damage and ultimate C exhaustion, a number of control mechanisms are incorporated in the C system. In addition to the C3b inactivator, there are serum proteins which inactivate C1 (**C1 esterase inhibitor**) and the anaphylactic fragments C3a and C5a (**anaphylatoxin inactivator**); additionally, the *membrane-binding sites* on newly cleaved C component fragments are *short-lived* and some of the active *complexes* formed are *quickly dissociated*.

LYMPHOID TISSUES

The lymphoid tissues are a *two-tiered system* designed for *lymphocyte programming* and *mobilizing (mobil-*

ize = to assemble and make ready for use): 1, the central *lymphoid tissues*; 2, the *peripheral (secondary) lymphoid tissues*.

Central lymphoid tissues These are the lymphocyte *programming* organs.

Thymus Lies in upper part of chest; large at birth, progressively declines in size after puberty; receives unprogrammed lymphocytes from haematopoietic tissues and *programmes* them to become *resident thymocytes (thymus cells)* or *migrating T-cells* (i.e. *thymus-derived lymphocytes*). T-cells become long-lived circulating lymphocytes in blood and lymph and are mobilized in certain areas of the *secondary lymphoid tissues*. *Thymectomy (ectomy* = cutting out) in the newborn mouse leads to absence of T-cells in the circulation and secondary lymphoid organs.

T-cell, *characteristics* and *functions* Microscopically a small lymphocyte; in the mouse identified by certain *cell membrane Ags (surface markers)* such as thy-l, present on resident thymocytes and migrating T-cells, and *thymic leukaemia antigen* (TLA), present only on thymocytes. Sheep red blood cells will spontaneously cluster around human T-cells to form *rosettes*, this phenomenon being used for indentification. T-cells are the *effector* cells (i.e. produce certain effects) in *delayed hypersensitivity (DH)*, rushing to the site of DH reaction to release *lymphokines*; other T-cell *subsets* are defined on the basis of variability of function:

Helper T-cell (T_h) Helps B-cells to respond to *T-dependent* Ags.

Suppressor T-cell (T_s) Suppresses B-cell ability to respond to Ag.

Cytotoxic T-cell Destroys other cells (infected self cells, tumour and allogeneic cells) under certain conditions, but mechanism of action is not understood.

In both mice and men, these T-cell subsets can be identified by the possession of certain surface Ags peculiar to each subset; in mice known as Ly (lymphocyte) Ags, in man by several nomenclatures.

Bursa of Fabricius *(birds)*/**mammalian equivalent** In the *bird* a well-defined organ located at the anal end of the gut; physically absent in *mammals*, but functionally present in imprecisely defined *equivalents* (probably the *bone marrow*). Receives unprogrammed lymphocytes from haematopoietic tissues and *programmes* them to become *B-cells* (bursa, or *bone marrow, derived* lymphocytes); B-cells form minority population (ca. 25%) of circulating lymphocytes and are mobilized in defined areas of the secondary lymphoid tissues. Removal of bursa *(bursectomy)* from newly hatched chicks leads to absence of B-cells in circulation and secondary lymphoid organs.

B-cell, *characteristics* and *functions* Microscopically a small lymphocyte. Surface marker Ags are *immunoglobulin* in nature: *initially* IgM, often associated with IgD, *switching* to IgG, IgA or IgE as the B-cell develops; has cell surface *receptors* for Ab *Fc* and for *C3b*. Its function is the production of circulating Ig, partly directly, but mainly through conversion to *plasma cell* after Ag stimulation.

Plasma cell Paradoxically, *not* found in plasma but in tissues; develops from Ag-stimulated B-cell to produce and secrete Ab.

Secondary lymphoid tissues The lymphocyte *mobilizing* organs; it is in these organs that the IR is largely generated and controlled.

Spleen An abdominal organ, roughly organized into two areas—the *red pulp* and the *white pulp*—on the basis of their visual appearance; *T-cells* are largely mobilized in the white pulp, *B cells* in the red pulp, where *plasma cells* are also found. *Sessile Mϕs* and dendritic cells abound and (especially the latter) readily take up circulating Ags; lymphocytes leave and return via the blood stream.

Lymph nodes Found in fully developed form only in mammals; primitive forms in some other vertebrates; located in every corner of body to *drain lymph* from surrounding areas, *mobilizing* lymphocytes and *monitoring* for antigens. Architecturally divided into marginal area called the **cortex,** underlying **paracortical area,** and central **medulla.** *T-cells* are largely mobilized in the paracortical area, *B-cells* are mobilized in

quiescent clusters (**lymphoid follicles**) in the cortex, while the *medulla* may show many *plasma cells* after antigen stimulation. Antigen stimulation also converts the lymphoid follicles into active **germinal centres:** collections of activated *lymphocytes,* many undergoing *blast* formation, together with *plasma cells* and *Mϕs; sessile Mϕs* and dendritic cells abound. Lymphocytes enter the node mainly through the walls of the post-capillary venules, which have an unusual structure, the endothelial lining being tall *cuboidal* rather than flat *squamous* (*squama* = scale)—hence *high endothelial venules.* The cuboidal endothelial cells may possess certain surface features recognized by lymphocytes prior to entry into the node. Lymphocytes leave via **efferent** (*ex* = from) lymphatic vessels. The extracellular fluid (which may contain Ag) passes to the node via **afferent** lymphatics (*ad* = to), and particulate matter is filtered out by the phagocytic activity of sessile Mϕs; soluble Ags may enter the Mϕs for processing via *pinocytosis.*

GALT and **BALT** Intimately associated with the gut epithelium and lungs, are lymph-node-like structures named respectively *gut-associated lymphoid tissue* (**GALT**) and *bronchial-associated lymphoid tissue* (**BALT**). Major *function* seems to be to supply IgA secreting B-cells and plasma cells to the local tissues.

Lymphocyte traffic Lymphocytes divide their time between the lymphoid organs and the bloodstream; normally, relatively few lymphocytes enter the somatic (*soma* = body) tissues on *routine policing duty.* In particular circumstances (e.g. *delayed hypersensitivity*

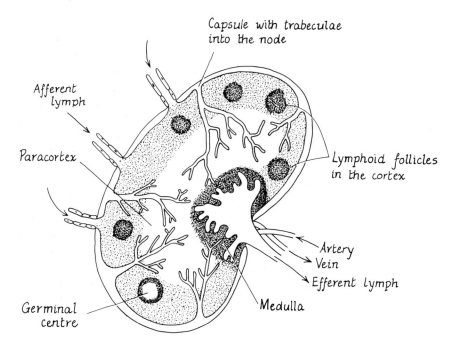

Figure 16. Lymph node structure, with division into cortex, paracortex and medulla.

reaction, *intracellular infection*) they leave the capillaries in large number and invade the tissues; in *granulomas* they may actually organize themselves, together with MΦs, into **local lymphoid organs**.

Thoracic duct The main 'link road' between the lymph nodes and the bloodstream, collecting the lymphocytes from the efferent lymphatic vessels and channelling them into the venous circulation.

NON-LYMPHOID TISSUES

Mast cells Strongly resemble basophils both in appearance and in function, but, unlike basophils, are resident in *tissues*. Large, blue-staining granules in cytoplasm contain pharmacologically active *mediators*, which are released in *anaphylactic* and *complement-fixing* IRCs to produce *inflammation*. Membrane has *receptors* for Fc region of IgE.

Capillaries Ultra-fine terminal blood vessels; walls are single layer of endothelial cells; become involved in immunological inflammation through activity of vaso-active amines released from basophils and mast cells. Local **stasis** (= standing still) of blood is produced by capillary dilatation; the capillary walls become more *permeable*, allowing *escape* of plasma and *selective migration* of leucocytes into local tissues; together this produces *reddening*, *oedema* and *cellular infiltration* of the tissues involved. The type of infiltrating cell depends on the nature of the chemotactic factors generated in the immunological reactions. Capillary walls may also become the sites of *deposition of immune complexes* with concomitant fixation and activation of C, again giving rise to *immunological inflammation*.

Smooth muscle Found in wall of *hollow organs* (*gut, bronchioles, uterus*); *contract* under the influence of mediators released by basophil/mast cell degranulation.

Sessile MΦ (*sessile* = sitting) MΦ which *sits in tissues*, particularly of the **reticuloendothelial system**: i.e. the network (*rete*) of phagocytes spread through the *spleen, lymphoid tissues, liver* and *bone marrow*; thus also known as the **mononuclear phagocyte system**.

Langerhans cells Ag-retaining and Ag-presenting cells, **dendritic** (= tree-like, i.e. branching) in form; found chiefly as network in the *epithelium* of the skin (ca. 1000 per mm^2)–hence, **reticuloepithelial system**.

Target tissues In certain situations almost any tissue or organ in the body may become the *target* (= something fired at) for immunological attack; the command which starts the firing is an *immunological reaction*, in the course of which *chemical mediators* are created or released; some of these mediators produce *inflammation* in the target tissue; others are *chemotactic* and cause a selective invasion of the tissues by WBCs; some mediators (e.g. *histamine*) are *preformed* within certain cells and are released in particular immunological reactions. Others (e.g. *bradykinin*) are *formed de novo* from precursors in the blood. Several situations in which immunologically-induced chemotaxis occurs are:

Infection When microorganisms invade a tissue to set up an infection, the cells brought to the site by chemotaxis may be seen to serve the teleological function of making the tissue *'safe'* by attacking and eliminating the invader.

Tumour surveillance The policing of the body cells by the WBCs to detect, attack and eliminate any cell which *mutates* to become cancerous before the mutated cell can multiply to the point of becoming an uncontrollable tumour. An attractively plausible teleological hypothesis in which the immune system again takes on the role of making the body safe, but which is now in disfavour for lack of convincing evidence.

In infection and tumour surveillance (if it indeed exists) the immune system can be seen to be serving its function by turning infected or cancerous tissues into targets and firing WBCs at them to eliminate the infection or cancer. Perplexing and/or vexing are other immunological situations, in which turning a tissue into a target for WBCs is seen to do harm, or, at best, no obvious good. Such situations are:

Hypersensitivity As previously defined, a situation in the living animal in which combination of Ag with IR products leads to inflammation with resultant cell or tissue damage; much of the damage may be produced by the WBCs brought to the target tissues by chemotaxis.

Autoimmunity A paradoxical term which, literally translated, means safety against self (*auto*); in fact, autoimmunity is just the *opposite*: an immunological situation in which the mechanism of self-recognition fails and the body mounts an attack on its own tissues (hence, more aptly termed **autoallergy**: an altered response to self). Though the primary immunological event may be humoral, chemotactic infiltration of WBCs is probably the major cause of tissue damage.

Graft rejection The damage and rejection of a grafted foreign tissue or organ (e.g. as in kidney transplant). The host's IR to the foreign donor HAs, and the subsequent IRC between the IR products and the foreign Ag, generates chemotaxis to produce invasion, damage and rejection of the grafted tissue. This is an immunologically sound, but pragmatically frustrating, situation.

2. Enter the Antigen

The single event which *triggers* the immunological chain is the arrival of Ag. Ag may arrive by several routes; experimentally or therapeutically it may be given with *adjuvant*.

Routes of entry Ag may gain entry into the body of its own accord, by self-administration, or through the manipulations of the clinician or immunologist.

Inhalation: *passage across the respiratory mucosa* Pollens, dusts, non-infectious microorganisms, experimental Ag.

Ingestion: *passage across the gastro-intestinal mucosa* Foods, drugs, experimental Ag.

Injection (also, **parenteral**): *directed penetration into the body* Secretions of biting or stinging insects, drugs (e.g. penicillin), other therapeutic substances (e.g. insulin), experimental Ag. Modes of injection include:

   intradermal (ID), intracutaneous (IC): *into the skin;*
   subcutaneous (SC): *between the skin and underlying structures;*
   intramuscular (IM): *within a muscle bundle;*
   intraperitoneal (IP): *into the peritoneal cavity;*
   intravenous (IV): *into a vein.*

Contact: *on skin or mucous membrane surface with subsequent chemical (covalent) bonding to tissue protein* Chemicals (e.g. dinitrochlorobenzene used experimentally); plant substances (e.g. poison ivy); drugs; metals (especially nickel); detergents; dyes and perfumes (as in cosmetics).

Infection: *Not really a route of entry, but a special situation in which the Ag gaining entry by any of the above routes is a disease-producing organism: Virus, bacterium, fungus, protozoan, metazoan.*

Transplantation *Organ or tissue transplant from one individual to another.*

Adjuvant (= *to help*) A substance which increases (**potentiates**) the IR induced by an Ag (hence, **immunopotentiation**). Action may be via *delayed absorption* (**depot effect**), by inducing *local inflammation* and *congregation* of lymphocytes and monocytes at Ag site (**granuloma formation**), or by some *undefined stimulus* to the immune system; some commonly used adjuvants:

Freund's incomplete adjuvant (FIA) A *water-in-oil emulsion*. The absorption of Ag from dispersed water droplets is retarded by a mineral oil barrier which makes up the continuous phase of the emulsion: i.e. a *depot effect*. Also: *granuloma formation*, possible *immune system stimulation* by mineral oil.

Freund's complete adjuvant (FCA) FIA with addition of *mycobacteria* to further stimulate immune system, possibly via enhancement of $M\phi$ *activity*.

BCG (Bacillus Calmette-Guérin) *Attenuated* form of *Mycobacterium tuberculosis*; same activity as mycobacteria in FCA.

Alum-precipitated antigen *Depot effect* obtained by adsorption of Ag to aluminium hydroxide formed by precipitation from alum. Retarded absorption plus granuloma formation.

Bordetella pertussis The whooping cough bacillus, usually referred to as **B. pertussis.** Killed organisms are a particularly effective adjuvant in rats and mice; *stimulates immune system.*

Endotoxins Cell-wall material from certain (gram-negative) bacteria; mode of action not completely understood, but $M\phi$s *are stimulated.*

Chemical nature of Ags Generally *polypeptides (proteins)* or *polysaccharides*; less commonly *polynucleotides (nucleic acids)* or *lipids*.

Synthetic Ags *Tailor-made molecules*, generally polypeptides built up from constituent amino acids; have been used to study the basis of immunogenicity.

Conjugated Ags *Chemical attachment* (= *conjugation*) of *haptens* to polypeptides and proteins to study the relative roles of *epitope* and *carrier* in the induction of an IR; also for purpose of producing Ab to hapten, particularly for *radioimmunoassay*.

Characteristics of Ags

Size A total molecular weight in thousands of daltons generally needed, varying with nature of the Ag; smaller molecules generally behave as *haptens*.

Hapten (= *to grasp*) A small molecule which in itself is not immunogenic, but *can bind* with (i.e. grasp) specific

Ab raised against an *epitope* of same structure; may be **monovalent** (binding with only one Ab molecule) or **multivalent** (binding with several Ab molecules). When *chemically conjugated* to a large molecule (**carrier**) the hapten itself becomes an **epitope** and acquires immunogenic potential from overall size of conjugate.

Foreignness (= *non-self*) Prescribed by necessity for avoidance of IR to self tissue and to prevent self-damage: what Ehrlich called '*horror autotoxicus*' (= *fear of self-poisoning*). But requirement is not absolute: exceptions—response to self Ags may pathologically occur spontaneously, or be induced by use of appropriate injection techniques. There are variable *degrees of foreignness*, the terminology for such often being ambiguous and varying in different situations.

Degrees of foreignness

Auto- = *self*, i.e. non-foreign; as in **autogenous** *(genous* = produced by), **autologous** *(logous* = relation), **autoantigens**; normally non-immunogenic, but bear in mind *autoimmunity*;

  Syn- = like, i.e. of the same genetic make-up.

  Allo- = other, i.e. Ags differing between (other) members of the same species; as in **alloantigens**; confusingly, *iso* = same (in the sense of being from the same species) is used synonymously in some situations, especially the **isoantigens** of the blood group systems.

  Hetero- = other, but '*more*' other, i.e. from another, or strange, species or source (hence also **xeno-** = stranger); therefore, the maximum degree of foreignness, as in **heterogenous, heterologous, heteroantigen, xenoantigen.**

  Sequestered Ags These are a special case: though really *autoantigens*, they lie *shut away* from direct access to the circulation; the lens of the eye is a good example. When nature, surgeon, or immunologist upsets their seclusion and they gain access to the lymphoid system, such Ags are *regarded as foreign* and induce an IR.

  Generally, the greater the degree of foreignness, the greater the immunogenicity of the Ag; on the other hand, to induce an IR to alloantigen, it is better to use a different member of the same species, rather than a member of another species. The latter would respond preferentially to species-specific heteroantigen, taking little note of the alloantigen; whereas to the former, Ag specific to its own species is autoantigen and is to be ignored. Therefore, it will respond to those alloantigens which are different from its own. A good example of this principle is blood group system Ag: a rabbit injected with human Rh+ RBCs would make essentially anti-human RBC Abs, while a Rh− human would make anti-Rh Ab. Abs to isoantigens are called **isoantibodies.**

Chemical configuration Regardless of size and foreignness, some substances are better Ags than others. This seems to be determined by the chemical building blocks from which the Ag is constructed and by the **tertiary structure** (shape) of the molecule. A synthetic polypeptide made from a single amino acid is less immunogenic than one made from a mixture of amino acids. Aromatic amino acids seem to give more immunogenic potential to protein or polypeptide than do aliphatic (non-aromatic) amino acids.

Anatomy of an antigen Though the whole Ag is generally large, only *small structures* and *shapes* on the molecule *determine* its Ag specificities—hence, **antigenic determinants**. Shorter and equally descriptive synonym is **epitope** (*epi* = on + *tope* = place): i.e. a small antigenically active place ('bump') on a large molecule. It is the epitope which is recognized by the receptor on the appropriate lymphocyte (**immune recognition**) and binds with the appropriate paratope of the specific Ab (**Ag–Ab binding**).

  Epitope size Of the order of 6–8 amino acids on a protein, 6–8 sugars on a polysaccharide.

  Epitope heterogeneity As the surface of a large molecule is thrown up into numerous 'bumps' of various shapes and sizes, not all epitopes on one Ag need be (in fact, generally are not) of similar structure—i.e. a single Ag generally has a **heterogeneous** (*geneous* = kind) *collection* of epitopes. In a humoral response to a single pure Ag, a *whole family of Abs* may be produced, each corresponding to a different kind of epitope on the Ag.

  Epitope specificity The demand for a *good fit* between an epitope 'bump' and the complementary 'hollow' of a lymphocyte receptor or Ab paratope *builds specificity* into the immune system. The demand for good fit rests on the nature of the forces which bind 'bump' and 'hollow' together; these can be seen at work in *epitope-paratope binding.*

  Ag–Ab (epitope-paratope) binding The *forces* involved in binding Ag epitope to Ab paratope are *physical*; **covalent** (= chemical) bonding is NOT involved. Consequently, Ag–Ab combination is *reversible* by such measures as changing pH, salt concentration (**ionic strength**), or temperature. The physical forces involved are *individually weak* and of *ultra-short range*. This makes good fit imperative and dictates specificity: epitope must get close enough to paratope and make large-area contact with it to bring sufficient of the weak binding forces into play to hold the large Ag and Ab molecules together. The forces involved are:

hydrogen bonding: tendency of H atom linked to O or N atom to latch onto a pair of electrons belonging to O or N atom on a nearby molecule;

ionic (Coulombic) forces: attraction between negative charge on one ionized molecule and positive charge on another;

Van der Waals forces: interaction between the outer electron clouds of an atom on one molecule and electron clouds on another molecule;

dipole forces: magnetic forces set up within molecules by the spinning electrons; magnetic poles of one molecule interact with opposite poles on another;

hydrophobic forces: attraction of hydrophobic (*hydro* = water + *phobic* = fear) groups on one molecule for the hydrophobic groups on another.

Ab affinity Fit between epitope and paratope is relative. It can be more or less good, bringing into play a greater or lesser number of physical bonds; thus the binding of Ag and Ab may be more or less firm. The *firmness of binding* is termed *affinity*: Ab making good fit and firm combination is said to be **high affinity Ab**, one making poorer fit and weaker combination is said to be **low affinity Ab**. Ab affinity can be measured.

Ag–Ab cross reactions Though specificity is the password of Ag–Ab interaction, at times it seems to break down: antiserum to Ag X may appear to cross the specificity barrier by reacting with Ag Y; this is termed a *cross-reaction*. It is less anomalous than it appears to be — there are two legitimate possibilities for its occurrence:

Similar epitopes Though two epitopes may not be identical, they may be sufficiently similar to allow a reasonable fit and a *more-or-less* good binding: the

identical reaction can be shown to be greater than the cross reaction (Fig. 17), because more perfect fit brings more binding forces into play and combination is less reversible — i.e. Ab has greater affinity for its own autologous epitope.

Shared epitopes Non-identical Ags may *share* one or more identical epitopes. Antiserum raised to either Ag will contain some Ab capable of binding with corresponding (shared) epitope on the other: again, the identical reaction will be quantitatively greater than the cross-reaction (Fig. 18); in this case because more Abs (anti-C, anti-D, anti-H, anti-S) are avail-

1. Antiserum A contains anti-S, anti-H, anti-D and anti-C:

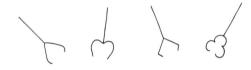

2. Antigen A possesses epitopes S, H, D and C, and reacts well with antiserum A:

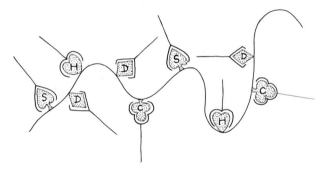

3. Antigen B possesses epitopes H, X, Y and Z and by nature of the shared epitope H, also reacts with antiserum A:

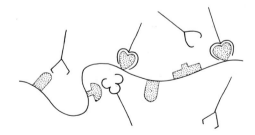

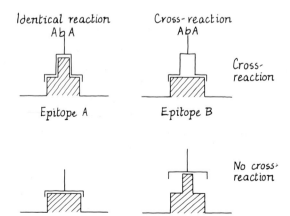

Figure 17. Cross-reaction due to similar epitopes.

Figure 18. Cross-reaction due to shared epitopes.

able for binding in the former than in the latter (anti-H only).

Fate of Ag

Soluble Ag Regardless of route of entry, soluble Ag quickly finds its way into the blood and/or lymphatic vessels; in addition to Ag in solution, this includes blood-borne viruses and soluble Ag released by infectious organisms. On its way round the body the Ag may meet various fates:

pinocytosis by motile Mφs, which may process it and/or present it to circulating lymphocytes;

pinocytosis by sessile Mφs and Langerhans cells, again possibly a preliminary step to presentation to lymphocytes;

direct contact with circulating lymphocytes (65–85% T-cells), which may then become mobilized in the lymphoid tissues;

entry into the lymphoid tissues to make contact with dendritic cells and the B and T lymphocytes mobilized there.

Particulate Ag A case of the mountain refusing to come to Mahomet, so the immune system comes to the Ag:

neutrophil: we cannot overlook the neutrophil: though no direct role in the *specific* IR is assigned to the neutrophil, it undoubtedly has an accessory role; being a phagocyte *par excellence*, it may be the *first* to arrive at a site of infection; one of its functions in this case *may be to take up* the particulate Ag, chew it up and then, in a mad suicidal act, destroy itself to *release* Ag in *soluble* form to the immune system;

lymphocyte: may invade the site of particulate Ag deposit and make *contact* with it; may then migrate to be mobilized in regional lymph node, or remain to participate in local granuloma formation;

Mφ: invades site and takes up Ag by *phagocytosis*; may leave site with Ag, or remain in local granuloma.

Role of the Mφ

In terms of initiating an IR, the Mφ, whether motile or sessile, may be the *key cell*. In its routine of phagocytosis and pinocytosis it ingests both particulate and soluble Ags; such Ag capture and subsequent processing may be the 'fuse' which ignites the IR 'powder'. There is good evidence that lymphocytes, at least in culture, fail to make a primary IR to many Ags in the absence of Mφs. The functions served by the Mφ in the IR are, as yet, ill-defined, but some credible probabilities are:

ingestion: taking up Ag via pinocytosis or phagocytosis;

fragmentation: this almost certainly is a prerequisite for particulate Ags; soluble Ags may be enzymatically degraded into small, perhaps epitopically less complex, fragments; this may be the first requirement for Ag processing;

concentration: packaging a lot of Ag in one parcel;

surface trapping: recycling phagocytosed, fragmented, concentrated Ag into its surface membrane, for

transportation and

presentation to the lymphocytes in *required form* and *concentration*; an absolute requirement for the response to most Ags; involves cell *contact* between Mφs and lymphocytes during which Ag comes into contact with *recognition receptors* on the lymphocyte; T-cells also require interaction with *compatible MHC Ags* on the presenting cells—this is known as *MHC restriction*; in some cases the Mφ secretes a *soluble factor*, containing Ag fragments and MHC products, which can present Ag to T-cells in the absence of Mφs—**genetically related factor**;

granuloma formation: collection at a site of particulate Ag deposit, together with lymphocytes, to form a lymphoid organ (*granuloma*), with all the required elements for producing a local IR.

The Processing Climax: 'All roads lead to Rome' and all Ag processing leads to confrontation between Ag and lymphocytes recognizing its epitopes; the lymphocyte may be a recognition B-cell or recognition T-cell. What happens next depends on a certain sequence of events.

Role of the Langerhans and dendritic cells

Like the Mφs, these cells seem to function as Ag-presenting cells in their respective sites. The Langerhans cells of the skin have the particular ability to convert simple chemical haptens into foreign epitopes on protein carrier molecules, thus rendering them immunogenic; therefore, they may play a primary role in *contact sensitivity*.

3. The Covert Immune Response

The processing step is essentially a *non-specific basic defence mechanism*. Almost everything that enters the body is subject to this preliminary 'going-over', particularly by the phagocytes. But it may also be the *prelude to an IR: the specific response to a specific challenge*. If the IR is switched on, activity first takes place, so to speak, behind the scenes: i.e., within the lymphoid tissues. This activity is not yet open or readily observed: basically, it can only be seen by microscopic examination of these tissues. In a word, it is *covert*.

THE IMMUNOLOGICAL INQUISITION

This could be dubbed 'the moment of truth': the point at which the body determines whether it can, or will, make an IR to a potential Ag. Not every invading substance, even if it has all the required characteristics of an Ag, will act as an immunogen. Before it can stimulate an IR, it must pass *three inquisitorial tests*.

1. Presence of immune response gene (Ir gene)

This is a gene which codes for a particular 'hollow' in a lymphocyte receptor or Ab paratope; if an Ag is to be effective, the body must have an Ir gene which produces a *recognition receptor* for one of its epitopes — otherwise there is nothing for the epitope to bind to and it goes unrecognized. In the case of T-dependent Ags, it may be a receptor on a T_h cell; there is also speculation that the Ir gene may dictate the manner in which the Mϕ handles a particular Ag. There is considerable evidence in *congenic animals* that the Ir genes are *located in the MHC*; evidence for Ir genes in humans has been difficult to obtain (because of the lack of inbred and congenic strains!), but can be inferred by the observed differences in humans in IR to the same Ag. Since epitope binding to lymphocyte receptor and/or Mϕ handling of Ag is the key to turning on the IR, no Ir gene means no IR; but, if the appropriate Ir gene for one or another epitope on the Ag is present, the Ag has passed the first test.

2. Acceptance as non-self

Self is determined during the ontogeny of the IR. Presence of Ag at the precise time (**'critical period'**) at which the immune system is due to acquire immune competence for that Ag has the effect of repressing the Ir genes relating to that Ag (so that no recognition clone is developed for it) and/or producing suppressor cells to it. Thereafter, the body will regard such Ag as self and refuse to respond to it. In the mouse and chick the critical period for most Ags coincides with *birth* or *hatching*, but in the sheep many Ags will only be recognized as self if present during a particular stage of *fetal life*. Since most self Ags (apart from the sequestered ones) will be circulating at the critical period for each, IR to them or any Ag strongly resembling them is just not on; so Ag of self origin, or accepted by the lymphoid system as self, will (bar exceptions) make no immunogenic impact; but, if an Ag is accepted as *non-self*, it has passed the second test.

3. Immunocompetence

In the final analysis, to make an IR the immune system must be *competent*; there are three situations — immunodeficiency, immunosuppression and immune tolerance — in which the immune system lacks this competence — i.e., it is immuno*incompetent*.

Immunodeficiency Refers broadly to conditions in which there is *defective functioning* of any part of the immune system; e.g. **congenital** (= *born with*) failure of development of some elements of the immune system, as in **thymic hypoplasia** (*hypo* = less; *plasia* = formation).

Immunosuppression This is a non-specific shut-down of the immune system which may occur *secondary* to some other disease process (e.g. in advanced stages of some cancers) or may be *induced* by the immunologist or physician in a variety of ways:

   chemical: by such drugs as cyclophosphamide, methotrexate, azathioprine; act by *interfering* with nucleic acid and protein synthesis, and so *inhibiting* cell division;

radiological: a high dose of X- or gamma-*radiation destroys* lymphoid tissues;

biologically: by injection of *antiserum* prepared against lymphocytes, or purified *Ab globulin* prepared from such antiserum—i.e. **anti-lymphocyte serum (ALS)**, or **anti-lymphocyte globulin (ALG)**; destroys lymphocytes, primarily T-cells;

surgical: *removal* of *bursa* in newly-hatched chick produces *B-cell deficiency; removal* of *thymus* in newly born mice produces *T-cell deficiency.*

Immune tolerance Blocking of immune competence to a *specific* immunogen: the immune system will tolerate the Ag and not make a response to it. It can be *induced* during ontogeny by injecting Ag at critical period, thus deceiving the immune system into accepting it as self Ag. May also be inducible in immunologically mature animal by using abnormally *high* or abnormally *low* doses (i.e. **tolerogenic doses**) of Ag:

low zone tolerance: tolerance is to *carrier*, rather than to **humorogenic** (= *Ab inducing*), epitopes—i.e. tolerance is induced in *T-cells*, which then produce T_s cells and/or fail to co-operate with the appropriate B-cells; tolerance can be *broken* by presenting the humorogenic epitope on a different carrier to which the body is not tolerant, thus bringing new sets of T_h cells into play and bypassing any T_s cells;

high zone tolerance: *both T-cells* and *B-cells* are made tolerant: receptors for both carrier and humorogenic epitopes are involved; in the case of the B-cells, may simply involve an overwhelming *blockade* of the receptors.

If the animal is not immunodeficient, immunosuppressed, or immunotolerant to the Ag, the Ag has successfully completed the immunological inquisition and the covert immune response goes into action.

LYMPHOCYTE STIMULATION

Getting back to our thesis of 'bumps' and 'hollows', everything which has taken place up to this point is simply to determine the existence of T-cells and B-cells with the right 'hollow' for recognizing the 'bumps' on the Ag; this is the corollary to our hypothesis of 'good fit'.

B-cell Ag receptor Simply an Ig molecule (generally IgM) on the cell surface; functionally it is a specific Ab with a paratope 'hollow' for one particular epitope 'bump'. All the immunoglobulin paratopes on one B-cell have identical epitope specificity—i.e. one B-cell can recognize only one specific epitope (always allowing for cross reactions). IgD is also found on many B-cells in association with IgM, but its function is not known; IgG, IgA and IgE are less commonly found as receptors on

B-cells. Thousands of *identical* Ag recognition receptors are present on one B cell.

T-cell receptor Evidence for Ag recognition receptors on T-cells is largely functional. While the T-cell is also specific in recognition of, and reaction with, Ag, the chemical nature of the receptor is unknown. T-cells have no detectable surface Ig. Further complexity has arisen from the discovery that T-cells recognize foreign Ag in association with self MHC Ags on presenting cells.

If the immune system is given the 'all clear', presentation of Ag to lymphocytes with appropriate receptors sets the immunological ball rolling. While events follow very similar lines in both B-cell and T-cell pathways the controlling factors and end results differ; both undergo transformation and mitosis and clonal expansion.

Transformation and **mitosis** The small lymphocyte manufactures much cytoplasm stuffed with RNA and *transforms* into a large *blast* cell (hence: **transformation, blast formation**). Since the cytoplasmic RNA in this large cell stains bright red with the dye *pyronin*, it also goes by the name **large pyroninophilic cell**. Blast formation is but a step towards *cell division* (**mitosis**: the blast cell duplicates the DNA in its nucleus, then divides to produce *two* daughter lymphocytes. Since the daughter cells arose from the original stimulated lymphocyte, they both carry Ag recognition receptors *identical* with that of their parent.

Clonal expansion The daughter cells are in turn transformed into blast cells, which then produce a second generation of *four* daughter cells, *and so on*, till the IR runs its course. The end result is *expansion* into a *family* of cells, all tracing their ancestry back to one original Ag-stimulated lymphocyte; such a family is called a **clone**. All the lymphocytes in one clone are identical twins in terms of type of cell (B or T) and of the Ag recognition receptor they carry: i.e. each recognizes precisely the same Ag epitope; but they may end up with *different* functional roles—just as one human identical twin may end up a parson, the other an immunologist.

T-cell pathway The role of the Mφ does not end with Ag presentation; initiation and maintenance of T-cell proliferation also requires the action of *intercellular* mediators, produced from Mφ and T-cells and known as **interleukins** (*inter* = between; *leukins* = produced by and acting on leucocytes). The result of transformation and clonal expansion of the T-cells is the production of **effector** cells which may mediate *delayed hypersensitivity*; express *cytotoxic* activity; *help* or *suppress* humoral responses; become *memory* cells.

B-cell pathway On stimulation, the B-cell becomes totally committed to the production of a humoral IR; therefore, the principal end cell of B-cell transformation and clonal expansion is the **plasma cell**—the *Ab factory*. In the response to most Ags the B-cell requires the *help* of a *(helper) T-cell*; Ags requiring T-cell help are called **thymus dependent** (= **T-dependent**) **antigens**. The phenomenon is known as **B-T-cell cooperation** and is achieved by the release of *soluble helper factors* from the T-cell, which provide a necessary stimulus to the B-cell. *Both IgM and IgG* are produced in response to *T-dependent Ag*.

T-independent Ags These are Ags to which the B-cell responds *without* T-cell cooperation; they are generally large polysaccharides with *many identical epitopes*. The Ab response is of *IgM class only*.

Ab responses to both T-dependent and T-independent Ag can be inhibited by T_s cells.

Some B-cells in the clone revert to small lymphocytes with an enhanced *memory* for the specific Ag—i.e. **memory B-cells**.

Three possible mechanisms of B-cell activation are postulated:

1. **Critical matrix theory** suggests that simple cross-linking of surface Ig (to form a *matrix*) is itself sufficient to trigger B-cell transformation.

2. **One signal theory** argues that the binding of Ag to the B-cell surface Ig is a passive event serving only to secure the Ag, which then imparts an activation signal to the B-cell by way of a separate '*activation receptor*'.

3. **Two signal theory** suggests that Ag binding to the surface Ig is a *first signal*; a *second signal* is required for full B-cell activation. The second signal is postulated to be supplied by *soluble factors* derived from helper T-cells. It has been further suggested that, if the Ag binds to the B-cell in the absence of the second signal, tolerance, rather than activation, results.

4. The Overt Immune Response and Immune Reaction

When the activity behind the scenes is completed, when the cells have gained their commitment to particular roles, the IR comes onto the stage, readily *open to view*: the **overt IR**. Whether humoral or cellular, primary or secondary, in the overt stage the IR can be shown to have taken place by means of an IRC between Ag and some product of the IR; such reaction may be observed *in vivo* or *in vitro*.

In vivo, the reaction may be observed in the animal which has made the IR, or in another animal to which the IR products have been passively transferred. Abs other than IgE can be passively transferred to and demonstrated in virtually any other animal; there is no strain or species restriction. IgE is restricted to the same, or closely allied, species by virtue of its *homocytotropic* nature.

By contrast, because of the MHC Ags they carry, study of passive *cellular immunity* by T-cell transfer is *generally restricted* to genetically identical animals: i.e. an identical twin, or another individual of an inbred strain. To avoid uncertainty over which cells are responsible for the IRC, the host lymphocytes may be destroyed by irradiation before transfer of the donor lymphocytes. Since the transferred lymphocytes are then 'adopted' by the recipient, the process is termed **adoptive transfer**.

The first meeting of Ag and immune system, in which memory plays no part, is a *primary response*; subsequent meetings, featured by the participation of memory cells, produce a *secondary response*.

Primary IR Because the immune system has no forewarning, its ability to respond to a *first (primary) exposure* to an Ag is limited: the primary IR is *slow* in onset, taking around 7–10 days to reach appreciable heights or to reject a first-set skin graft; is of *low* magnitude, as measured by Ab levels; and of *short* duration, waning in a matter of weeks. In the humoral response *IgM is predominant*, with a subsidiary IgG response. To many Ags (T-dependent Ags) *immunological memory* is established, so that subsequent exposure to these Ags results in secondary IR.

Secondary IR The memory cells left behind from the primary IR act like a *booster* rocket to send the IR off into 'orbit' (hence, **booster dose; booster response**). Onset is *fast*, being demonstrable in 2–4 days, magnitude is *high* and duration is *long*, often persisting for years. IgG now predominates in the humoral IR; therefore, IR to T-independent Ags, which induce only IgM, lacks memory. Since *memory* is at the root of the secondary IR, it is also referred to as the **anamnestic** (= *memory*, *recall*) response.

HUMORAL IMMUNE RESPONSE

The end result of B-lymphocyte stimulation by Ag is Ab production. How is specificity of the Ab achieved? Two opposing theories have been proposed to account for this specificity.

Instructive theory suggested that Ag *instructed* the cell to produce specific Ab by itself acting as a **template** (= *pattern*) on which the Ab was *directly* folded in complementary shape (**direct template hypothesis**), or by modifying the DNA or RNA in which Ig was coded (**indirect template hypothesis**). Now discredited and replaced by selective theory.

Selective theory Each B-cell possesses membrane Abs of *one predetermined specificity*. The specificity of the membrane Ab is determined by the selective expression in the cell nucleus of only one gene coding for a V_H and another for a V_L, the combination producing an Fab paratope recognizing a specific epitope. When Ag arrives it *selects* those B-cells carrying membrane Ab with paratopes corresponding to one or another of the Ag epitopes, these cells alone undergoing transformation and *clonal expansion* (hence also, **clonal selection hypothesis** of Burnet). Two theories have been put forward to account for the *total range* of Ab specificities (the **Ab repertoire**):

germ line theory proposes that the Ab repertoire will have been arrived at by *evolutionary mutation* of Ab-coding genes in the ancestral germ cells (*germ line genes*); doubt has been cast on whether there are sufficient germ line genes to account for the seemingly vast repertoire of Ab specificities, giving rise to the:

somatic mutation theory, which contends that germ line genes must be supplemented by **somatic** (*soma* = body) mutation in the lymphocyte genes during lymphocyte ontogeny.

The *potentials* of the humoral IR in terms of IRC—including the teleological one of fighting off infectious agents and their products—are determined by the classes and subclasses of Ab produced: there are five classes (with subclasses) of Ab.

IgM

The *first* Ab to appear after Ag stimulation and the third most abundant in serum; almost exclusively a **pentamer**—i.e. compounded of five (= *penta*) parts (= *meros*), each part being a **monomer** made up of two μH chains and two L chains. The five monomers are joined together at the C-terminal ends of their H chains by *inter-chain -S-S- bridges* (Fig. 19), the formation of these bridges being initiated by the attachment of a **J** (= joining) **chain** to one of the H chains; thus a big molecule (mol wt. 900,000, sedimentation constant 19S—hence, **macroglobulin** and **19S Ab**). The J chain (15,000) is synthesized in the same plasma cell as the Ab; theoretically IgM has a valency of 10 (i.e. should bind 10 identical epitopes, as it has 5×2 paratopes), but practically the valency depends on the size of the Ag. Usually the valency is about 5 because the crowding of five Ags around the corona of paratopes makes a solid (= *steric*) barrier which hinders the approach of additional Ags: so referred to as **steric hindrance**. Multivalency increases the functional **affinity** (= strength) of binding between Ag and Ab; this is beneficial because various functions secondary to binding Ag are achieved more effectively by higher affinity Ab. IgM has no memory, the secondary response showing the same characteristics as the primary response; therefore, a raised IgM titre is generally indicative of an ongoing or recent infection; distinctive for IgM are:

> *immediate activation of classical C pathway:* immune complexes containing IgM are especially effective in fixing C1q because of the intrinsic high Fc density;
> *powerful agglutination of particulate Ags* because of multivalency.

Natural antibodies Abs present in serum directed against Ag not known to have been previously encountered are usually IgM: e.g. isoantibodies against A and B blood group Ags, which are probably produced as IR to cross-reactive Ag from gut bacteria.

IgG

The historically classical Ab; predominant Ig in serum, comprising 75% of total serum Ig; a monomer consisting of two γ H chains and two L chains, held together by -S-S- bridges, producing two paratopes and generally a valency of 2 (= **divalent**); mol wt. 160,000, sedimentation constant = 7S. 4 subclasses based on structural differences in the γ chain and numbers and positions of interchain bridges: IgG1, IgG2, IgG3, IgG4, which also have functional differences; passes readily into the tissues from the circulation because of its relatively small size. IgG is notable in the following areas.

Memory It is the form in which B-cell (humoral) memory is expressed, rising dramatically in secondary IR.

Placental transport Crosses the placenta from mother to fetus in many mammals to provide essential *passive protection* to the immunologically immature neonate; may, however, have harmful result, as in *haemolytic disease of the newborn*, in which IgG Abs directed against *Rhesus* (Rh) blood group Ag pass from Rh-negative (Rh−) mother to Rh-positive (Rh+) fetus, resulting in C-activated destruction of fetal RBC.

Activates (except IgG4) classical C pathway on interaction with Ag. IgG4 fails to fix C, possibly because rigidity in hinge region covers C1q binding sites. As monomer, is intrinsically not as effective as IgM in C-activation, but, especially after secondary IR, overtakes this inferiority by sheer molecular numbers.

Precipitates soluble Ag Particularly effective and important because of high serum IgG titres obtainable; together with C activating property, results in *Arthus*

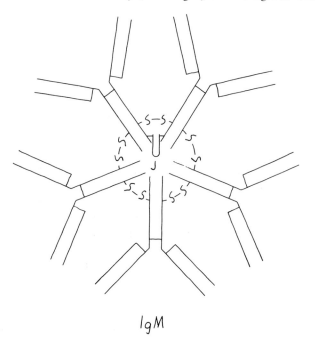

IgM

Figure 19. IgM.

reaction on local administration of Ag.

Agglutinates particulate Ag Again, *vis-a-vis* IgM, makes up in quantity its valency inferiority. Binding with failure to agglutinate occurs in certain situations: unfavourable positioning of Ags on particle surface, rigidity of Ab hinge region (= **incomplete Ab**). Notably encountered in *Rh blood group testing*, in which low density and rigid fixation of Rh Ag on RBC surface results in *failure of agglutination* of Rh+ cells in presence of anti-Rh. Non-agglutination in this circumstance is overcome by adding *albumin*, which decreases repulsive forces between the cells, so requiring less cross-linking by Ab, or by agglutinating the Ab-coated cells with *anti-IgG Ab* (= **Coombs' test**).

Opsonin Particles (e.g. cells) coated with IgG become more susceptible to phagocytosis by macrophages (IgG1 and 3 only) and neutrophils (IgG1, 2, 3, 4). This activity is potentiated by C fixation, since C3b allows binding of particles to phagocytes with C3b receptors.

Antibody-dependent cell-mediated cytotoxicity (ADCC) The non-specific killing of IgG-coated target cells by *K cells* with Fcγ receptors.

Neutralizes (i.e. renders ineffective) toxins and viruses; in the latter case entry into host cells is prevented.

Heterocytotropic Ab Ab that binds via Fc to receptors on mast cells and basophils of some other (= *hetero*) species more effectively than to cells of the species of origin — e.g. *rabbit IgG* binds better to guinea-pig cells than to rabbit cells. Subsequent encounter between Ab-coated mast cell or basophil and Ag results in *anaphylactic degranulation;* transfer of such Ab from an immunized animal to a non-immunized animal to produce mast cell/basophil sensitivity to Ag is called **passive sensitization,** commonly carried out experimentally in skin, when it is termed **passive cutaneous anaphylaxis (PCA).**

IgA

A dual purpose Ab: second most abundant Ig in serum and major Ig in external secretions — mucus, colostrum, tears, saliva, sweat; 2 subclasses, IgA1 and IgA2. An interesting allotype of IgA2 exists, with no L-H interchain -S-S- bridges; instead, the molecule is stabilized by L-L -S-S- bonds and interacting physical forces.

Serum IgA

90% IgA1, 10% IgA2; more than 80% in *monomeric form*; mol wt. 160,000, 7S; some in *dimer form* (mol wt. 350,000, 9S) in association with a *J chain* structurally identical to that found in IgM. No established secondary effector functions, which may be beneficial in that IgA could damp down the inflammatory changes triggered by IgG and IgM (C fixation, anaphylaxis, chemotaxis) by competing for the Ag. In *aggregated* form, IgA may activate C by alternate pathway.

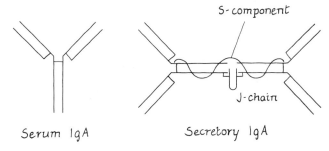

Figure 20.

Secretory IgA

Produced by local plasma cells in mucosal tissues: e.g. gut, respiratory tract; 50% IgA1, 50% IgA2. Exists predominantly as a *dimer* (mol wt. 400,000; 11S) with *J chain* and **secretory component (SC,** mol wt. 60,000), the latter produced by the mucosal epithelial cells. On leaving the submucosal plasma cells and entering the overlying epithelium, the dimeric IgA picks up the SC, which then promotes active transport of the secretory IgA across the epithelium and onto the mucosal surface. SC stabilizes the molecule and makes it *resistant to proteolytic digestion*—very important in the gut.

Properties of secretory IgA

Bacterial lysis In association with *C* and *lysozyme*, an enzyme present in tears, nasal secretions and on the skin.

Inhibits bacterial attachment to epithelial surfaces and prevents *colonization*, e.g. is protective against caries formation by *Strep. mutans*.

Antiviral activity High *neutralizing* Ab titres in the secretions confer resistance to viruses which usually enter via surfaces protected by these secretions; e.g. oral polio vaccine raises intestinal IgA anti-polio Ab and is far more effective in producing immunity than any other route of administration.

Maternal IgA Ab in the colostrum provides important gut protection to the neonate.

IgD

Little known because it is present in minimal quantities

in serum (0–0.3 mg/ml); studies with IgD *myeloma proteins* suggest that its mol wt. is 185,000 with 4 constant domains in the δ chain; 7S; no Ab activity demonstrated in normal serum. It is a major *B-cell surface Ig*, found on 70% of peripheral B-cells with IgM; its roles in the serum or on cell surfaces remain unknown.

IgE

Present in smallest quantity in serum (20–450 ng/ml); monomer, mol wt. 200,000; 8S; 4 constant domains in the C chain; heat labile.

Properties of IgE

Homocytotropic Ab ('reagin') Ab that binds via Fc preferentially to cells of the *same species*; especially refers to binding to *mast cells* and *basophils*, such that subsequent interaction with Ag causes *degranulation* of those cells, with the release of *vasoactive mediators* (Fig. 21) such as *histamine, prostaglandins, slow reacting substance of anaphylaxis (SRS-A)* and *chemotactic agents* (e.g. *ECF-A*). These mediators produce *anaphylaxis* or a *Type I hypersensitivity reaction*; raised levels of IgE are thus found in *atopic* individuals i.e. those with an inherited tendency to develop Type I hypersensitivity.

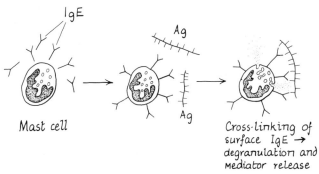

Figure 21.

'Gatekeeper' effect An inflammatory change (i.e. *increased capillary permeability*) that occurs when an Ag interacts with mast cell-fixed IgE; allows infiltration into the area of other classes of Ig which can neutralize, fix complement, and opsonize. IgE thus acts as a **gatekeeper,** opening the capillary wall *'gates'* to release Ab-containing plasma and phagocytes, augmenting the battle against invading foreign organisms.

Anthelminthic IgE levels are raised in individuals infected with *helminths* (worms); IgE's protective value results from the release of mediators which themselves produce an unfavourable environment and cause infiltration of *eosinophils* into the area. Eosinophils have been shown to be involved in the destruction of helminths.

Heat labile Destroyed by heating at 56°C for 1–4 hours; a distinguishing characteristic.

CELLULAR IMMUNE RESPONSE

The cellular IR includes those responses which do not require the participation of Ab and which can be transferred from an immune to a non-immune individual by activated lymphocytes, the central cell being the *T-cell*. It is the T-cell which determines *specificity, memory* and *transferability* in the cellular IR. The end result of the blastogenesis and mitosis following T-cell activation by Ag is the production of **effector** (= effect producing) T-cells and the release of soluble mediators (named **lymphokines** by Dumonde).

Effector T-cells come in several categories, identifiable both by the presence of certain *surface Ags* and by their **effector functions** (the effects they produce on reaction with Ag). These functions may concern immune attack or immune regulation. In either case, the effector cells generally interact only with other cells (lymphoid or non-lymphoid) which carry the same ('self') MHC Ags: hence, **self restriction.**

Cytotoxic T-cell (T_{cyt}) Destroyer of infected cells, allogeneic cells and, possibly, cancer cells. Destruction of cell wall of cells harbouring infective agents (viral, bacterial, fungal or protozoal) exposes the agent to Ab and phagocytes; in the case of allogeneic cells, as in graft rejection, the T_{cyt} recognize the foreign MHC Ags and attack the cells carrying them. Though definitive evidence is lacking, in some instances T_{cyt} are capable of killing tumour cells *in vitro,* suggesting a possible role for these cells in **tumour surveillance:** the watchful *surveying* of the body by the immune system to identify and destroy tumour cells as they arise. Supporting evidence for immune surveillance is sparse, since the hunt for tumour-specific Ags has so far been largely inconclusive.

Helper T-cell (T_h) Has the function of prodding B-cell to mount an IR against T-dependent Ags; the T_h recognizes Ag epitopes different from those recognized by the B-cell.

Suppressor T-cell (T_s) Like the T_h, recognizes specific Ag epitope, to which it responds by suppressing the B-cell response to humorogenic epitopes. One vital suppressor function may concern induction of tolerance to self tissue; another could be that of regulatory mechanism for shutting down the IR when it has done its job.

Lymphokines (*kine* = move) are non-Ab glyco-proteins which act as intercellular mediators of the cellular IR; large numbers have been identified and classified mainly by their activity in vitro; important examples are:

Mø chemotactic factor: lures Møs into the area of a cellular immune reaction;

Mø migration inhibition factor (MIF): *inhibits the migration* of Møs, thus localizing them at the site of lymphocyte activation;

Mø activating factor (MAF): may be identical with MIF; *activates* the localized Møs to enhanced phago-cytic, bactericidal and tumoricidal function; activation is non-specific, the Møs killing unrelated organisms as well; localized and activated Møs are the weapons of cell-mediated immunity against many intracellular infections, emphasizing the role of lymphokines in the immune defence mechanism;

mitogenic factor: causes transformation and *mitosis* in non-committed 'bystander' lymphocytes, releasing more lymphokines and augmenting the cellular re-sponse, demonstrating a possible *amplification role* for lymphokines;

lymphotoxin (= a toxin derived from lymphocytes): can by itself produce lysis of cells in the absence of lymphocytes;

skin reactive factor (SRF): a lymphokine whose activity is demonstrated in vivo; when injected into skin, it causes *increased capillary dilatation and permeability*, resulting in **erythema** (= redness) and **induration** (= hardening), the latter due to fluid and cellular infiltration of the site; like many lymphokines, the chemical nature of SRF is unknown and this inflammatory activity may be carried out by a number of lymphocyte release products acting collectively;

interferon: a much publicized substance because of its supposed anti-tumour effect; it is released in different forms during viral infections from a variety of cell types, including lymphocytes and activated Møs; all forms have in common the ability to *prevent viral replication* within cells and it has consequently been suggested that interferon plays a major role in protection against viral infections; it also stimulates NK cells, which then show increased tumoricidal activity.

IMMUNOTECHNOLOGY

The existence of IRC has enabled immunology to build up a detection and assay technology all its own, but one which has been avidly adopted by every other biological science because of its specificity and sensitivity. For *large*

molecules it is without parallel; and for many small molecules of biological interest, conjugating the *small molecule* to a macromolecular carrier makes the use of immunotechnology equally available.

Some immunotechnology is inherent in the immune system itself—primarily the mixed lymphocyte reac-tion; but mostly it is grounded on the fact that IR leads to immune products which will, in turn, react specifically with the original inducing Ag. Add to this the ingenious array of reaction indicators—fluorescein, ^{125}I, horse-radish peroxidase, ferritin, to name but a few—which immunologists have mobilized for visualizing and/or increasing detection sensitivity and ease of assay, and immunotechnology can rival or outperform most com-peting technologies.

Immunotechnology has expanded so much, it now commands do-it-yourself books in its own right. So, for our present purposes, we need but look at a few basic or representative immunotechniques. These can be divided into two groups: one based on the *humoral* response (Ab), the other on the *cellular* response (effector T-cells).

Humoral immunotechnology

Precipitation (Kraus)

Basically, Ab will precipitate with soluble Ag. For decades precipitation was carried out in the fluid state in tubes, purely as a gross technique for identifying 'Ag' (usually a mixture of Ags—e.g. from a bacterium) and 'Ab' (actually, a corresponding mixture of Abs). With this technique it was possible to tell human serum from goat serum, grass pollen from tree pollen, one micro-organism from another. One could diagnose infections, classify and sub-classify microorganisms on the basis of their antigenic differences and similarities, and separate out Ags and Abs from mixtures, when one or the other was available in pure form; but it was not possible to compare directly and discriminate between several Ags or Abs in mixtures, because they all came down together in *one cloud of precipitate*.

Through the ingenuity of Oudin, Oakley & Ful-thorpe, Elek and Ouchterlony, plus the innovative talents of other immunologists, a whole repertoire of discriminative precipitation techniques have been devised on the principle of immunodiffusion.

Immunodiffusion (Oudin; Oakley & Fulthorpe) A process whereby Ag and/or Ab are permitted to *diffuse* through a supporting gel (now generally agar) to form a visible, discrete band of precipitate where the Ag and Ab overlap in optimal proportions. The stabilizing of each Ag/Ab precipitate as a discrete band in the semi-solid supporting gel permits discrimination between different Ag/Ab systems. Originally carried out in tubes (Oudin; Oakley & Fulthorpe), but now replaced by agar plates in the following modifications.

Double diffusion (Ouchterlony; Elek) Generally referred to as the Ouchterlony plate, though Elek published more or less simultaneously. Agar plates are poured and wells cut in the agar; Ag and Ab are placed in opposing wells; *both* Ag and Ab *diffuse* through the agar (= *double diffusion*) and eventually overlap. Since different Ag molecules in a mixture will generally be of different size, and since the Ag:Ab ratios for the different reactants will generally vary, the individual

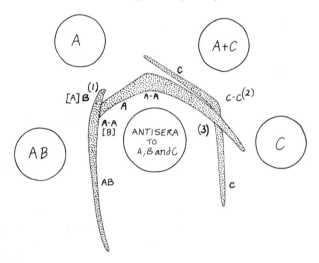

Schematic diagram of precipitation lines from a double immunodiffusion plate.

(1) Spur = reaction of partial identity
(2) Fusion = reaction of identity
(3) Cross-over = reaction of non-identity
A = Ag carrying epitope A
AB = Ag carrying epitope A and epitope B
C = Ag carrying epitope C

The antiserum contains Ab's to epitopes A, B and C

A[B] = Ag AB combining with Ab to A

[A]B = Ag AB combining with Ab to B, this Ab not being held back at A-anti A precipitation zone.

Figure 22.

Ags in the mixture will usually form *separate precipitation lines* with their respective Abs. When Ags are placed in separate, adjacent wells opposing the same Ab

well, the precipitation lines for the individual Ags, forming at their respective wells, will ultimately run into each other as they grow in length. If the Ags from the two wells are of completely different specificities (= *non-identical*), their precipitation lines will be uninfluenced by each other and simply cross (= **reaction of non-identity**); if the Ags from the two wells have *identical specificities*, they form a single pool of identical Ag molecules where they overlap and their individual precipitation lines will fuse into a smooth connecting arc (= **reaction of identity**). When the two Ags share some epitopes in common, but differ in other epitopes (i.e. are only *partially* similar), their precipitation lines will form a smooth arc, demonstrating the common epitopes, but a *spur* will go off on a tangent on one or both sides of the arc, demonstrating the non-identical epitopes (= **reaction of partial identity**)—always assuming that Abs are present for all the relevant epitopes. Thus, double diffusion proved a powerful *qualitative* tool, but showed little scope for quantitation.

Single radial immunodiffusion (Feinberg; Tomasi & Zigelbaum) This is a quantitative adaptation of immunodiffusion. Ab is mixed with the agar and Ag is placed in wells cut in the Ab-agar gel. As the Ag diffuses into the Ab-laden agar, a ring of precipitate is formed. At equilibrium (or at a fixed time), the diameters of the rings are proportional to the log of the concentration of Ag. Plotting the ring diameters of three known Ag concentrations on semi-log paper gives a straight line, from which the concentrations of test Ags can be assayed from the diameters of the precipitation rings they form. This technique is widely used in path labs for the assay of serum protein levels; unfortunately, it is often mistakenly referred to as the 'Mancini' technique.

Mancini technique Those who wish to carry out the *true* Mancini technique should proceed as for single radial immunodiffusion; when the precipitation rings have formed, the plate is placed in a photographic enlarger, 'the magnified rings are projected on strong paper and their contours pencilled out. . . . *The circles are cut out and weighed.*'

Immunoelectrophoresis (Grabar & Williams) As the name implies, *electrophoresis* and *IRC* (in the form of *immunodiffusion*) are combined. A protein solution (usually blood plasma in the hospital) is placed in a well in an agar gel on a slide or plate; a positive electrical charge is applied to one end, a negative charge to the other, sending an electric current through the gel. As the proteins carry charges on their amino (positive) and carboxy (negative) groups, they are carried (= *phoresis*) along the gel by the current; since the net charge may differ from protein to protein, different proteins will travel at different speeds and so separate along the length of the gel (*first separation*). At a suitable point, the *current is turned off* and antiserum is placed in a slot cut in the gel parallel to the direction of the electric current; now the proteins and antibodies diffuse freely through the gel and immunodiffusion precipitation bands are formed across the width of the gel (*second separation*) between the electrophoretic path and the antiserum slot. The position of each of the bands is unique, and constant in relationship to each other, thus allowing initial identification by running in parallel with a reference protein, and subsequent identification based on acquired familiarity with the precipitation pattern. Though essentially a qualitative technique, a quasi-quantitative assessment of protein concentration can be made by comparing the density of a precipitation band with that of a normal control—i.e. hypergamma-globulinaemia and hypogammaglobulinaemia can generally be spotted by running a patient's serum alongside a normal serum and comparing the densities of the Ig bands.

Modifications of immunoelectrophoresis:
    rocket immunoelectrophoresis (Laurell);
    immunoelectrophoresis on cellulose acetate (Kohn);
    cross-over (countercurrent) immunoelectrophoresis (Bussard);
    two-dimensional immunoelectrophoresis (Ressler; Laurell).

Agglutination (Gruber & Durham) C-inactivated IgG and IgM Abs to cell surface Ags will cross-link particulate Ags, causing them to stick together (= *ag-glutinare*) and produce aggregates, which can be detected macroscopically or microscopically. Used initially for the identification and study of micro-organisms, later for blood grouping, by specificity of their *intrinsic* (self) cell wall Ags. Subsequently, techniques have been developed for attachment of *extrinsic* (non-self) Ags to particulate carriers, extending agglutination to soluble Ags (= **passive agglutination**).

Indirect agglutination (Moreschi; Coombs) Some Abs (e.g. anti-Rh) will bind to Ag on cell, but are incapable of cross-linking the cells to produce agglutination (= **incomplete Abs**); in such cases, use of a second Ab specific for the first Ab, which is now cell-bound, will effect cross-linking and agglutination.

Complement fixation; complement lysis (Pfeiffer) In the presence of C, IgG and IgM Abs will lyse cells; if the cell is a bacterium, C lysis is observed as a clearing of the cloudy bacterial suspension; if it is a RBC, lysis is observed by the release of haemoglobin from the lysed RBCs. Released haemoglobin can be estimated by eye (*50% haemolysis endpoint*), or more accurately and sensitively assayed by measurement in a colorimeter. C lysis can also be accomplished by fixing of soluble Ag to RBC and mixing with specific Ab; alternatively, fixation of C in non-lytic Ag/Ab systems can be measured by using sensitized (= Ab-coated) RBCs as indicators of C depletion.

Labelled Ab immunotechniques In many situations it is useful to be able to visualize Ag/Ab interactions, or to increase the sensitivity of detection. Techniques have been devised for conjugating (*labelling*) Abs with agents which make this possible. The more prominent methods are:

immunofluorescence (Coons): Ab is labelled with a fluorescent dye; when the Ab binds to Ag the reaction can be visualized in situ by activating the fluorescent dye with UV light; primarily used to detect Ags on cells and in tissues;

enzyme-linked immunosorbent assay (ELISA) (Engval; Perlmann): Ab is labelled with an *enzyme* (horse-radish peroxidase; alkaline phosphatase; *et al*); for assay of bound Ab, the enzyme substrate is added to the system after the Ag/Ab reaction is complete; enzyme action on the substrate produces a coloured product, which can be assayed in a colorimeter as a measure of the amount of Ab bound; alternatively, the enzyme may be linked to the Ag; in either case, an inhibition assay technique may be used, measuring the extent to which a test Ag inhibits the binding of the enzyme-linked reagent;

radioimmunoassay (RIA) (Yalow & Berson): labelling the Ab or Ag with a *radioactive element* (e.g. tritium, ^{125}I) produces an ultra-sensitive assay system, based on the ability of radiation measuring instruments (beta counter; gamma counter) to measure infinitesimal amounts of the radioactive element; otherwise, similar to ELISA.

Passive cutaneous anaphylaxis (PCA) (Ramsdell; Ovary) An *in vivo* humoral technique, in which the skin (= *cutis*) of an animal (usually a guinea pig) is used as the site for IRC. Serum from an immunized animal is injected into the skin of a normal animal to produce areas of *passive sensitization*; some hours later, the Ag and a blue dye (Evans Blue; Pontamine Sky Blue) are injected IV into the animal. When the Ag combines with the Ab fixed on mast cells in the skin of the passively sensitized sites, local *anaphylactic* reaction occurs, with release of mediators. Increased capillary permeability allows the blue dye, along with the blood plasma, to leak into the skin within one half-hour; the forenamed dyes are persistent and leak out of the blood vessels into the whole skin within hours, colouring the entire animal for weeks. Feinberg introduced the use of Coomassie Blue as a non-persistent dye which is excreted within a few hours, leaving the animal colourless.

Pinnal anaphylaxis (Feinberg) An *in vivo* technique in which the ears (= *pinnae*) of animals (generally mice) are used as the site for Ag/Ab reaction, again utilizing a blue dye to visualize the IRC. Animals may be actively (systemically) sensitized, or the ears may be passively sensitized by local subcutaneous injection of an active serum. Challenge is by placing a droplet of Ag solution on the ear and passing a hypodermic needle through the droplet and on through the ear. Once again, local infiltration of blue dye at the site of challenge indicates an *anaphylactic* reaction.

Hybridoma technology, monoclonal Abs, T-cell markers

As the name implies, a hybridoma is a *hybrid* (= derived from different sources, one source being a tumour = *oma*). Actually, it is a hybrid produced by the fusion of a *terminal plasma cell* from an immunized spleen and an *eternal plasma cell* from a plasmacytoma (myeloma). From the former, the hybridoma inherits genetic information for the production of a specific Ab, from the latter it inherits eternal life and continuous productivity. The objective is to produce a single clone of perpetually dividing plasma cells, continually churning out a monoclonal Ab of desired specificity. Each cell in such a clone manufactures and exports Ab molecules identical in structure and epitope specificity—i.e. of identical isotype, allotype, idiotype—to those of every other cell in the clone.

Fusion is induced biologically or chemically by the technique of Milstein and Kohler. The cells are cultured in a medium in which unfused cells are eliminated. The hybridoma cells are initially binucleate, hence tetraploid, but they spontaneously lose chromosomes until they get down to the normal complement.

As can be expected, hybridization is a hit-and-miss proposition, any one of the spleen's myriad plasma cells being capable of fusing with the monoclonal plasmacytoma cells. This creates a heterogenous collection of Ab producing cells. These must now be separated into individual cells by diluting them out, the clones obtained from each of these cells then being resolutely screened to find the one producing Ab of the desired specificity. Once so identified, the clone can be used for continuous in vitro production of this monoclonal Ab.

Such Abs have proved to be of immense value. They have distinct advantages over polyclonal Ab prepar-

ations made by simple immunization of animals. Firstly, because all the Abs are of identical structure, they provide a source of homogenous material for detailed structural analysis of different classes and sub-classes of Ig, with the advantage over myeloma proteins that, as the epitope specificity of the monoclonal Ab is known, the structure and a.a. sequence of the paratope can be related directly to its specificity.

Secondly, since monoclonal Abs can theoretically be produced to any epitope, they provide a means of (a) separating one particular Ag from another and (b) identifying the presence or absence of a particular epitope on, for example, a cell membrane Ag. Indeed, it is in the sphere of cell surface analysis that they have made a major contribution to immunological studies.

Using monoclonal Abs, it is now possible to correlate the presence of certain lymphocyte membrane markers with the different functional lymphocyte sub-sets. This is most clearly defined for T-cell subsets in mice. The Ags involved were formerly designated Lyt(Ly = lymphocyte; t = T-cell), but are now more simply referred to as Ly Ags. There are three Ly Ags, designated Ly-1, Ly-2, Ly-3. Ninety-five per cent of thymocytes (that is, developing T-cells) possess all three Ly Ags: Ly-1,2,3. Similarly, 60% of circulating T-cells are Ly-1,2,3, while 30% are Ly-1 and 10% are Ly-2,3 (the Ly-2 and 3 Ags always occurring together). The Ly-1 cells include helper T-cells and T-cells responsible for delayed hypersensitivity reactions; Ly-2,3 cells include cytotoxic and suppressor T-cells. At least some of the circulating Ly-1,2,3 cells appear to be concerned with the induction and regulation of the IR.

In man, a similar system of T-cell surface markers has been identified by monoclonal Abs and variously (and confusingly) designated. A commonly used nomenclature is the OKT system (O = Ortho, the manufacturer of this line of monoclonal Abs; K = Kung, one of their scientists; T = T-cell). All the peripheral T-cells possess the markers known as OKT1 and OKT3. Helper T-cells have, in addition, OKT4 (equivalent to mouse Ly-1), while cytotoxic and suppressor cells are OKT5/8. During their development T-cells possess numerous other OKT Ags, which disappear or become undetectable with the maturation of the cell.

It is now less certain than was once believed that these T-cell markers correlate strictly with the functional T-cell subsets. Also, it is important to note that some of these markers are found on other cell types.

In fairness, it should be pointed out that an alternative form of nomenclature for human T-cell markers is the Leu system (Becton Dickinson), in which Leu-3 is identified on T_h and Leu-2 on T_s cells.

If all this diversity of nomenclature begins to sound alarming, harking (or turning) back to our discussion of cell membrane Ags in the section on 'The Cell' will bring matters into perspective.

Cellular immunotechnology

Mφ migration inhibition test If mononuclear cells (lymphocytes and Mφ) are packed into capillary tubes and cultured overnight in medium in a plate, the Mφ will migrate out of the tube, fanning out over the bottom of the plate. However, if Ag to which the T-cells are sensitive is added, the release of *MIF* prevents this migration, the extent to which it is *inhibited* giving an indication of the degree of sensitivity to that Ag.

Lymphocyte transformation test When sensitized T-cells encounter the particular Ag to which they are sensitive, they respond by undergoing *transformation* and mitosis, during which they manufacture new DNA. In the lymphocyte transformation test the synthesis of DNA is measured by culturing the lymphocytes with Ag in the presence of *tritiated thymidine*. After several days of culture, the amount of radioactive thymidine taken up by the cells is measured with a *β-counter*: this gives an indication of the amount of DNA synthesized and, hence, of the degree of sensitivity to the Ag. This technique is also used to study in more detail the chemical events in lymphocyte activation: in this case instead of using an Ag to stimulate specific clones of cells, substances known as **mitogens** (= stimulators of mitosis) are used. These stimulate cells *non-specifically*, i.e. their action is not restricted by Ag specificity. Consequently, the number of cells stimulated is very large and the events occurring are far more easily measured: some mitogens are selective for T-cells (e.g. *phytohaemagglutinin*), some for B-cells (e.g. *pokeweed mitogen*).

Mixed lymphocyte reaction (MLR) When *lymphocytes* from two individuals are *mixed* in culture they respond to the *foreign MHC Ags* on each others' cells by transforming and dividing, a *reaction* which can again be assessed by measuring tritiated thymidine uptake. In this case, the activity measured reflects the proliferative activity of both sets of lymphocytes—**two-way MLR**. In a **one-way MLR**, one set of lymphocytes is prevented from responding by treating it with *X-rays* or *mitomycin C*, an antimitotic drug; thus the response of only one set of cells is recorded. The antigenic determinants responsible for stimulating proliferation are the *lymphocyte activating determinants (LADs)*. The degree of proliferation thus reflects the degree of genetic disparity between the two individuals. Since these LADs are among the Ags recognized by the host immune system on a transplanted organ, MLRs between potential donors and recipient are performed prior to transplantation to determine the likelihood of rejection or acceptance of a graft: the MLRs (two-way and one-way in both directions) should be as low as possible, if the graft is to survive.

5. Mishaps of Immune Response and Immune Reaction

To take a leaf out of the book of Voltaire's Dr Pangloss, Nature clearly intended for its creatures that all should be for their best in this best of all possible worlds. Occasionally Man intends the same. But, to paraphrase Robert Burns, the best laid plans of Nature and Man often go astray.

The immune system is no exception: abnormalities, defects, eccentricities occur in the immune system of some individuals just as they do in other systems of the body. In some instances the by-product of a defence-oriented IR and IRC may be the inflammation and tissue damage of *hypersensitivity*; in others the immune system may turn against some body tissue to produce an *autoimmunity*; there are occasions of both *excessive* and *deficient* activity of one or more arms of the immune system; and all too frequently man's intention of replacing a damaged organ meets stern opposition from the immune system and the transplanted organ is *rejected*.

HYPERSENSITIVITY

A situation in the living animal in which combination of Ag with IR products leads to *inflammation* and *damage* of cells or tissues; classified by Gell and Coombs into *four types*, designated by Roman numerals; Types I–III are Ab-mediated, Type IV cell-mediated.

Type I hypersensitivity

Also known as *anaphylactic* or *immediate* hypersensitivity. Ag combines with *mast cell-* or *basophil-fixed IgE; degranulation* of these cells occurs with release of mediators: histamine, chemotactic factors, prostaglandins, leukotrienes, 5-hydroxytryptamine, platelet activating factor. There follows *increased capillary dilatation* and *permeability* with leakage of plasma into the tissue — **oedema formation** (oedema = swelling); if this reaction occurs in the *skin*, it is visible as *reddening* and *swelling* at the site — **wheal and flare reaction**. These changes are noticeable within 10–15 minutes (hence known as **'immediate'**), reach a maximum at about 30 minutes and then slowly fade. If the reaction occurs in the lung, these mediators have the effect of *constricting the bronchi*, resulting in increased resistance due to narrowing of the airways, producing difficulty in breathing.

Anaphylaxis

The term anaphylaxis dates from work by Richet and Portier in 1902. These workers showed that injection of an Ag into animals that had been previously sensitized to that Ag caused the development of an extremely severe systemic reaction, involving a drop in blood pressure and asphyxia, which was in many cases fatal. Injection of the same Ag into unsensitized animals had no adverse effect. They therefore concluded that the initial exposure had rendered the animals unprotected and named the phenomenon **'anaphylaxis'** (*ana* = lack of; *phylaxis* = protection). This word is a misnomer, since we now know that the condition is not principally a passive loss of protection but *is in fact* an actual infliction of a state of sensitivity. While some of the chemical mediators responsible for this effect were subsequently uncovered fairly rapidly, the exact mechanisms involved in anaphylactic or Type I hypersensitivity have only been elucidated in the last two or three decades.

Histamine A derivative of the aromatic amino acid, *histidine*; it is *preformed* in the mast cell or basophil granules, ready to be released. It is a potent *vasodilator* and *increaser of capillary permeability*; consequently it can itself produce a **wheal and flare** reaction — i.e., oedema surrounded by reddening — when injected into the skin; *contracts smooth muscle* in, for example, bronchi, uterus, gut.

5-Hydroxytryptamine (5-HT) A derivative of the amino acid tryptophan, 5-HT is found in large quantities in *human platelets* and in the mast cells of other species, e.g. the rat. It *constricts larger vessels, increases capillary permeability* and *contracts smooth muscle*.

Prostaglandins A series of related compounds, named from A to I according to slight differences in structure, with subscripts to indicate the number of —C$=$C— double bonds e.g. PGE_1, PGI_2, PGD_2. They are all derivatives of the unsaturated fatty acid *arachidonic acid*, which is produced from membrane *phospholipids* when the cell is appropriately stimulated—i.e. these PGs are not preformed. PGD_2 is released from *mast cells* and *basophils* during *anaphylactic reactions*; it causes *smooth muscle contraction* and is a *vasodilator*.

Leukotrienes A class of compounds also derived from *arachidonic* acid, but by the action of a slightly different enzyme; individually named LTA_4 (an unstable intermediate), LTB_4, LTC_4, LTD_4, and LTE_4, these substances are many times more *potent* than histamine at *increasing capillary dilatation* and *permeability*. **Slow reacting substance of anaphylaxis (SRS-A)** is in fact a mixture of certain leukotrienes released from mast cells and basophils during anaphylactic reactions; it causes a *contraction of smooth muscle* that is *slow in onset* (hence, *slow reacting*) and of long duration.

Platelet activating factor (PAF) also not preformed, being generated on stimulation of the cell; it *causes platelets to release vasoactive amines*.

Eosinophil chemotactic factor of anaphylaxis (ECF-A) *Attracts eosinophils* to the site of a Type I reaction; the eosinophil's role is not understood but it has been suggested that it may act to limit the tissue damage by releasing *inactivators* of histamine, SRS-A, and PAF.

Neutrophil chemotactic factor of anaphylaxis (NCF-A) Neutrophils are also attracted to the site, but substances which simply increase capillary permeability will also promote escape of circulating neutrophils into the tissue.

In addition to these release products of mast cells and basophils, **bradykinin** (*brady* = slow; *kinin* = action) also becomes involved in Type I reactions. It is a *nonapeptide* (*nona* = nine) produced from a plasma protein precursor, *bradykininogen*. The conversion is brought about by the action of *kininogenases* produced during the course of a Type I reaction; bradykinin is a *more potent vasodilator* and *increaser of permeability* than histamine, but *acts more slowly*. It can also increase pain sensations.

Anaphylaxis can be *local* (degranulation of mast cells in a particular tissue), or *general* when mediators are released from *basophils* in the circulation and/or mast cells throughout the body. In this latter case the drop in blood pressure (**hypotension**) and *bronchial constriction* can be severe enough to cause death. Fortunately, general anaphylaxis is not common but can occur in certain hypersensitive individuals in response to drugs such as penicillin; *local anaphylactic* reactions, on the other hand, are common: **hay fever** (sensitivity to grass pollens), **asthma** (= panting) and **urticaria** (= nettle

rash; *urtica* = nettle) are familiar manifestations of Type I hypersensitivity; occurring in *atopic individuals*, generally referred to as *allergies* in clinical situations.

Atopy The hereditary predisposition to develop Type I hypersensitivity; approximately *15–20%* of the population are *atopic*.

Allergies may be treated by **chemotherapeutic** (*chemo* = chemical) or **immunological** means. Chemotherapeutic agents include *antihistamines*, which prevent the inflammatory action of histamine, and drugs which prevent mast cell and basophil degranulation, such as *disodium cromoglycate*. The immunological approach is to *hyposensitize*.

Hyposensitization (*hypo* = lower) This consists of administering over a period of time *graded doses* of the Ag to which the individual is hypersensitive; this prevents or reduces the development of anaphylaxis on subsequent exposure to the Ag. It has been suggested that this procedure acts by raising the levels of *IgG Ab* to the Ag; this IgG (known as **blocking Ab**) combines with the Ag, blocking its access to the basophil or mast cell fixed IgE.

Type II hypersensitivity—cytotoxic/cytolytic hypersensitivity

Mediated by *IgG* or *IgM* Ab directed against Ags on the surface of cells; these Ags may normally be a part of the cell (**intrinsic**), or may be small molecules which have become *covalently* attached to the cell (**extrinsic**). Destruction of the cell can occur by several mechanisms:

C activation: both IgG and IgM attached to Ag fix C by the classical pathway, with eventual cytolysis by the terminal components, C8 and C9;

opsonization: IgG and C3b can opsonize the cell for ingestion by Mφs or neutrophils;

ADCC: again IgG mediated, killing being achieved by cells with receptors for Ab Fc (K cells, Mφs, neutrophils) and which can thus treat Ab-coated cells as targets.

These mechanisms of killing are normal, essential features of defence against a wide variety of invading organisms. Tissue damage and hence Type II hypersensitivity occurs when the Abs are directed against Ags on self cells or on transfused RBCs. The following are important clinical examples.

Rhesus incompatibility When a Rh− mother (one whose RBCs do not possess Rh Ags) bears a Rh+ child, some of the child's RBCs may pass into the maternal circulation during parturition. The mother will then produce Ab against Rh Ags; if she then carries another Rh+ child, this Ab, usually IgG, will cross the placenta and react with the fetal RBCs, with resultant lysis: **haemolytic disease of the newborn**.

Autoimmune haemolytic anaemia A disease in which an IR is set up against certain intrinsic RBC Ags. This results in lysis of the RBCs (hence **haemolytic**) and consequently **anaemia** (= no blood).

Drug reactions Certain drugs will combine *covalently* with cells in the body; Ab directed against these *extrinsic Ags* will cause cytolysis, e.g. *phenacetin* binds to RBCs inducing Ab to the drug, which then causes **drug-induced haemolytic anaemia**; *amidopyrine* binds to granulocytes to similarly produce **agranulocytosis**; *sedormid* can cause destruction of platelets in the same manner.

Blood transfusion reactions Any person possesses, in his plasma, *IgM natural Abs* against ABO blood group Ags which are not present on his own cells; these have arisen from contact with *cross-reacting Ags* on gut bacteria. If someone is transfused with *mismatched blood* (i.e. containing foreign ABO Ags) these natural Abs recognize and react with the transfused cells; *C activation* occurs throughout the body and not only results in destruction of the foreign RBCs, but also in *general anaphylaxis* (due to the anaphylotoxins, C3a and C5a), *aggregation of platelets (disseminated intravascular coagulation)* and, if severe, *renal failure* due to the fall in blood pressure. These effects may be evident within one to two hours of transfusion and, if they develop, the transfusion should be stopped immediately.

Blood grouping and crossmatching

Red blood cells, like all other cells, possess Ags in their cell membrane. These RBC Ags, which act as surface markers, have been classified into a number of systems; ABO, Lewis, Rhesus, Kell, Duffy, etc. The most important, and the first to be described (by Landsteiner in 1901), is the ABO system. The *ABO Ags* are in the form of *glycolipids*, the *lipid* moiety being embedded in the membrane and forming the basic structure to which certain *sugar residues* are attached. It is these sugars that impart the antigenic specificity. The simplest Ag in this system is known as H substance; the attachment of the sugar residue *N-acetyl galactosamine* to H substance produces *A substance*, while addition of *galactose* gives rise to *B substance*. The addition of these extra residues is under the control of transferase enzymes coded for by *'a'* and *'b' genes* respectively. While some individuals have neither of these genes and do not convert H substance to either A or B substance, others may be homozygous for 'a' or 'b' genes, or heterozygous,

carrying one 'a' and one 'b' gene. On this basis, and as the genes are co-dominant, their RBCs will exhibit A, B or A and B Ags respectively. Thus, individuals are grouped in the following manner:

Antigen	Blood group	% of UK population
A	A	43
B	B	9
A and B	AB	3
Neither (i.e. just H substance)	O	45

Group A, B and AB individuals also possess a small amount of unconverted H substance on their membranes.

A further important aspect of the ABO system is that people's serum contains *natural IgM Abs* directed against Ags not found on their own RBCs; this is extremely important when it is necessary to transfuse blood from one individual to another, as is frequently the case in hospital practice. If, for example, group B blood is transfused into a group A patient, the latter's natural anti-B Abs will destroy the donor RBCs and give rise to a *transfusion reaction*, in which there is massive C activation, RBC destruction and a generalized anaphylaxis that can be fatal. Consequently, it is essential to know the blood group of both *donor* and *recipient* prior to transfusion; this is achieved by a simple haemagglutination test in which the 'unknown' RBCs are mixed on slides with Abs of known specificities. Haemagglutination then indicates the presence of the particular RBC Ag against which the Ab is directed and thus identifies that individual's blood group.

Group O blood possesses no Ags that are not present on other people's cells and can be transfused to an individual of any blood group without the danger of a transfusion reaction; hence, group O individuals are known as *universal donors*. The corollary to this is that since group AB individuals possess A, B and H substances they will not have Abs directed against any of these and can therefore receive any group of blood—hence, *universal recipients*.

Also of importance in practice is the *Rhesus* system of Ags. This system consists of a number of *protein Ags*, the most important of which (because of its high immunogenicity) is called the *D Ag*. People with D Ag on their red cells (85% of the Caucasian population) are traditionally known as Rh+. Unlike the ABO system, individuals without the D Ag (Rh−) do not possess natural IgM anti-D in their serum, but rapidly develop a mainly IgG anti-D response if they are given Rh+ blood; subsequent administration of Rh+ blood can lead to a marked transfusion reaction. A similar situation exists in haemolytic disease of the newborn, but in this case the mother has developed anti-D in response to fetal Rh+ cells which entered her body at a previous birth.

For safety reasons, blood of the same ABO and Rh D groups is used for transfusion whenever possible. However, in an emergency, when there is insufficient time to determine the patient's blood groups, group O Rh− blood carries the least danger of inducing a reaction.

If more precise information about the compatibility of a particular donor and recipient pair is required, *cross matching* can be performed. This involves mixing the blood donor's RBCs with the recipient's serum (in saline at room temperature to identify the IgM Abs and in albumin at 37°C to demonstrate IgG Abs). The absence of haemagglutination indicates that the recipient does not possess Abs against donor cells and, therefore, that no transfusion reaction will develop, while agglutination indicates that a reaction will occur, and transfusion of that recipient with that donor's blood should be avoided. Cross matching has the advantage over simple ABO and Rh blood grouping in that it also demonstrates compatibility or not, as the case may be, at other blood group Ag loci. This is especially important when the recipient has already had multiple transfusions and is likely to be sensitized to many of the lesser RBC Ags.

Type III hypersensitivity — immune complex mediated

Also known as *late* or *intermediate*; IgG and/or IgM complexes are formed and activate C; the complexes may be retained *locally* or *circulate in the bloodstream*, depending on the Ag:Ab ratio. The response to products of C activation may lead to damaging inflammation — hence, hypersensitivity. Locally (e.g. in the skin), the reaction comes on in 3–6 hours — hence, **late** or **intermediate reaction**.

Circulating complexes When a large quantity of foreign Ag is injected into the bloodstream (e.g. when immune serum prepared in horses, such as antitoxins, is used to transfer immunity passively to humans) a humoral IR will be induced over a period of days; as Ab appears, immune complexes are formed in *Ag excess*. These are *soluble* complexes and circulate in the bloodstream. Initially small immune complexes are produced which are not deposited, not phagocytosed and are probably filtered by the kidneys; as Ab levels rise, large immune complexes are formed which are rapidly phagocytosed and again are not deposited. Problems arise in conditions of *mild Ag excess* when *soluble immune complexes* of *intermediate size* are produced; being neither removed by the kidney nor by phagocytosis, they are deposited in blood vessel walls. Deposition requires some prior alteration in blood flow in the region, which may result from C activation in the circulation, leading to histamine release from basophils through C3a and C5a activity.

When the complexes are lodged in the walls, C activation occurs and neutrophils are attracted to the site by the *chemotactic action* of *C5a*. These neutrophils attempt to remove the immune complexes and in the process release lysosomal enzymes into the area, causing extensive tissue damage. A further component is the activation and aggregation of platelets: this can cause vascular occlusion and ultimately **necrosis** (*necros* = dead).

Frequent sites of deposition are the *kidney, joints* and the *dermal-epidermal junction* in the skin. The term applied to the ensuing inflammatory changes (kidney lesions, fever, joint swelling, enlarged lymph nodes, urticaria) is **serum sickness,** developing several days after injection of, for example, a *heterologous antitoxin.*

Local complexes — Arthus reaction This is a local reaction elicited when an Ag enters the body of someone with high levels of *precipitating Ab*. The immune complexes formed in *Ab excess* precipitate out in the vessels at the site of Ag entry; with C activation and neutrophil infiltration, an intense local inflammatory reaction follows, reaching a peak 3–6 hours after contact with the Ag. Clinical examples of this can be seen in **extrinsic allergic alveolitis** (allergic inflammation of the alveoli due to foreign Ag), a term covering a multitude of conditions such as *bird fancier's lung* and *farmer's lung*. They are due to Type III reactions to inhaled Ag and are characterized by attacks of breathlessness some hours after contact with the Ag.

Type IV hypersensitivity—cell-mediated

A *cell-mediated reaction* also known as **delayed hypersensitivity (DH)** since it develops 24–48 hours after encountering the Ag. The damage is mediated by the interaction of Ag with *primed T-cells*, which then release *lymphokines*. These produce local changes in *capillary permeability* and *dilatation* and cause *infiltration* of the area by *mononuclear cells*; the recruited lymphocytes secrete more lymphokines and the Mφs may release enzymes capable of destroying surrounding cells, thus exacerbating the inflammation. If these events occur in the skin (e.g. on injection of Ag intradermally), the site becomes **indurated** (= hardened), due to the fluid and cellular infiltrate, and **erythematous** (= red).

The presence of DH to an intradermal injection of an organism is sometimes used to demonstrate immunity to that organism; for example, in the *tuberculin test* Ag extracted from *Mycobacterium tuberculosis* (**Purified Protein Derivative = PPD**) is injected and the site examined at 24–48 hours. The development of a DH reaction is usually taken to indicate protection against tuberculosis, provided there is no evidence that the patient actually has the disease. Absence of reaction is taken to indicate a lack of cellular immunity to TB and the advisability of vaccination with **BCG**, which is an *attenuated* form of the mycobacterium. In fact, DH and cell-mediated protection do not always correlate and can occur separately to the same Ag.

Contact sensitivity An inflammatory reaction in the *skin* that can occur on *contact* with a variety of external agents to which the body has become sensitized; it is caused by a DH reaction. While a number of small chemical compounds can act as sensitizers, they have in common the ability to *conjugate covalently* with *autologous skin proteins* (thus acting as *foreign epitopes* on the *conjugated Ag*).

On repeated exposure to such a compound DH develops, after which further contact causes inflammation. Nickel (e.g. necklace clasps), various topically applied drugs (e.g. neomycin) and compounds found in paints, dyes, detergents, cosmetics, toiletries, etc. are common sensitizers. Immunologists commonly paint *dinitrochlorobenzene (DNCB)* or *picryl chloride* onto the skins of animals to induce experimental DH.

AUTOIMMUNITY

During embryological development a 'pact' is signed which ensures that the immune system will not attack the rest of the body (or itself for that matter)—that is, a state of *tolerance* exists between the immune system and the body cells around it. Unfortunately, in some cases the deal comes with no guarantee, or the guarantee runs out too soon; self-tolerance then no longer applies and an IR can develop against self cells: **autoimmunity** (*auto* = self). When autoimmunity causes tissue damage, an **autoimmune disease** results; so autoimmune diseases are those diseases in which the damage present is a direct consequence of an *IR*, with subsequent *IRC*, *against self*. In most cases the factors causing the development of autoimmunity in an individual are poorly understood; this may be largely due to the lack of knowledge about the maintenance of self-tolerance in the first place; for example, it is clear that, if an Ag is presented to the immune system at a particular period of embryological development, it is regarded as self—i.e. the immune system is tolerant to it; however, what is not clear are the cellular events involved; there are two major propositions:

Clonal deletion This suggests that the clones capable of reacting with self are irreversibly eliminated during ontogeny; this neglects the fact that autoimmunity can develop at a later date and, therefore, the clones must be present. Consequently, this concept has been modified to **clonal inactivation**: i.e., the self-clones are inactivated, but not deleted.

Suppressor T-cells It is possible that Ab production against self Ag is held in check by suppressor T-cells; indeed, in some autoimmune diseases a precipitous loss of these cells does appear to precede the development of the disease, but the events leading to this loss are not known.

Autoimmunity can occur *spontaneously* or can, for the purpose of experimentation, be *induced* by immunizing with the Ag in question in *Freund's complete adjuvant*; this latter technique has provided useful animal models for a number of human autoimmune diseases.

Autoimmune diseases can be crudely classified into two categories: *organ specific* and *non-organ specific*.

Organ specific diseases

In organ specific diseases the IR and IRC are directed against Ag found only in one particular organ; important clinical examples are:

Autoimmune thyroiditis, in which Ab (mainly IgG, sometimes IgM) directed against a number of Ags in the thyroid gland (thyroglobulin, microsomal Ag) are suggested to be the direct cause of the inflammation and damage to the gland.

Graves' disease, also affecting the thyroid, but in which IgG Abs are directed against the receptor for *thyroid stimulating hormone (TSH)*. Rather than damaging these cells, they stimulate them to such an extent that too much thyroid hormone is produced (**thyrotoxicosis**), with numerous detrimental effects in the rest of the body; the Ab which binds with the receptor is known as **LATS** (= **Long Acting Thyroid Stimulator**) or **Thyroid Stimulating Ig** (= **TSI**).

Myasthenia gravis (*myo* = muscle; *asthenia* = weakness), a disease characterized by generalized muscle fatiguability which can be so severe that even respiratory muscles may be weakened. The defect lies at the *neuromuscular junction*—that is the point at which the nerve supplying a muscle meets the muscle; at this junction a chemical, *acetylcholine*, is released and acts on a *receptor* on the muscle to cause contraction. In myasthenia gravis, IgG Ab against this receptor is present and is directly responsible for the symptoms of this disease.

Non-organ specific diseases

An IR against Ag present throughout the body occurs in these diseases.

Systemic lupus erythematosus (SLE) Characterized by **antinuclear Ab (ANA)**: Ab to various constituents of cell nuclei such as DNA, RNA and nucleoproteins. These ANAs are responsible for the lesions in SLE. The damage is caused by the deposition of immune complexes containing ANA and nuclear Ag in various vessel walls, notably in the glomeruli of the kidney (causing **glomerulonephritis**) and at the dermal-epidermal junction in the skin. At this latter site the fixation of C and subsequent inflammatory changes cause the *erythema* which gives the disease its name. It should be emphasized that the Abs do not penetrate cells easily to react with, for example, DNA in the nucleus, but rather with nuclear Ag which has escaped into the circulation, hence the deposition of immune complexes in tissues.

Rheumatoid arthritis (RA) The major finding in this disease is the presence of Abs against the Fc portion of IgG molecules: these Abs are mainly IgM class, but can also be IgG. This gives rise to IgM-IgG and IgG-IgG immune complexes, which become deposited in the synovia of the joints. The subsequent inflammation leads to an influx of neutrophils with release of damaging enzymes: the area becomes inflamed, cartilage is broken down, and the joint becomes swollen and painful. Proliferation of cells lining the joint (possibly stimulated by *lymphokines*) causes further disruption of the area. Since these changes are a result of Abs directed against self IgG, the demonstration of these Abs in a patient's serum is a diagnostic test for RA.

Other autoimmune diseases

In addition to these two broad categories of autoimmune diseases there are some diseases in which IR against non-organ specific Ag appears, but in which only one organ is damaged; the classical example is *primary biliary cirrhosis*, in which anti-mitochondrial Abs are demonstrable. However, while mitochondria are essential constituents of all cells, the disease only affects the liver, with destruction of bile ducts.

Treatment

Treatment of autoimmune diseases includes several alternatives: in many cases, especially the severe ones, it is necessary to give *cytotoxic drugs* such as *cyclophosphamide* to kill the rapidly dividing lymphocytes. The problem with this approach is that the drugs are nonspecific in their action and the patient becomes *immunosuppressed* and consequently susceptible to infection. Another approach is to administer *steroids*: these have a number of effects on the immune system: both cellular and humoral IR are damped down, while neutrophil and $M\phi$ granules are stabilized, thus decreasing the release of damaging enzymes; the inflammation at the site of the autoimmune reaction is thus considerably reduced. However, steroids have numerous unpleasant side effects and prolonged use should be avoided, if possible. Finally, in many diseases the result of the attack on a particular organ may be a decrease (e.g. autoimmune thyroiditis) or an increase (e.g. Graves' disease) in production of a particular hormone; in such cases the correction of this imbalance does much to alleviate the symptoms of the disease.

GRAFT REJECTION

It has been man's dream for many years to treat a diseased organ by removing it and replacing it with a non-diseased organ. Indeed, it is into this area of **organ transplantation** that much human effort has been channelled. In most instances the technical difficulties of the surgical procedures have been surmounted; what is left facing the doctor (and the *transplanted organ*, or *graft*!) is the threat of the host's immune system. Since the organ is taken from another individual, genetic differences between *donor* and *recipient* exist (an exception is grafting between *identical twins*). These differences are recognized by the recipient's immune system and an IR is set up which is *generally cellular*, but may contain a humoral component. The subsequent IRC can cause so much damage to the graft that it no longer functions and is *rejected* by the recipient = **graft rejection**.

The Ags responsible for notifying the immune system that the graft is there are the LADs (Class II MHC Ags), coded for by the MHC; however, while these set the IR rolling, the Ags recognized as targets by both Ab and cytotoxic T-cells are the serologically determined Ags (Class I MHC Ags). Prior to transplantation, it is essential to perform **tissue typing** on the recipient and potential donors of the graft—i.e. to identify their MHC Ags; donor and recipient should be *matched* as completely as possible, if a graft is to survive. MLRs are also carried out and donor's and recipient's lymphocytes should stimulate each other as little as possible. Even when these precautions are taken, it is rarely possible to match completely and the presence of those remaining unmatched MHC Ags means that rejection can still occur.

Patterns of rejection As in any other IR, an accelerated rejection occurs on secondary exposure to a particular Ag on a graft: in transplantation immunology the terms **1st set rejection** and **2nd set rejection** are applied. Much of the information on the events occurring during rejection has come from studies of the numerous kidney transplants that are now being performed, and various modes of rejection have been described.

Hyperacute This can develop within minutes of transplantation and appears to be due to preexisting Ab against foreign blood group Ags, which will be present in a vascular graft.

Acute early developing in up to 10 days: the main feature is a dense cellular infiltration of the graft. The attack is cell-mediated involving both lymphokine release and T-cell cytotoxicity.

Acute late If the graft withstands the initial cellular onslaught, it may be open to attack by the developing humoral IR. Abs against MHC Ags cause the damage either through the activation of C or by acting as targets for ADCC.

Late rejection In the kidney this is associated with deposits of immune complexes in the glomerular basement membrane with subsequent damage to the kidney via C activation and neutrophil infiltration. The condition may arise either because of a previous immune complex disorder (i.e. a disease in which the damage is a direct consequence of the presence of immune complexes, e.g. SLE) or because Abs against soluble kidney Ags appear and become deposited in the forms of complexes.

Other methods of classifying rejection can be used (e.g. according to the type of cellular infiltrate), but the above readily demonstrates the wide variety of host defence mechanisms that the graft must withstand.

The doctor can come to the aid of the graft in a number of ways, all of which aim at compromising the host's immune system to a greater or lesser extent.

Azathioprine, a cytotoxic drug, has been used extensively since its introduction in the early 1960s. It hits rapidly dividing lymphocytes and also interferes with resting T-cells; its main effect is to prevent rejection crises and it has very little ability to abort a crisis once it has started.

Corticosteroids: prednisone is usually the steroid given. Often administered in addition to azathioprine, prednisone can be invaluable in reversing rejection crises once they have started.

Anti-lymphocyte serum (ALS) Used to deplete the recipient of lymphocytes, ALS is finding use as an accessory form of treatment in some cases.

Total lymphoid irradiation This was the mode of immunosuppression used in the early attempts at transplantation: it fell into disuse with the introduction of the cytotoxic drugs, but may be returning to favour.

Cyclosporin A Much interest has centred on this drug, which selectively interferes with T-cell activity; more information is required before an accurate appraisal of its capabilities can be made.

The major problem with all of these approaches is that they result in *immunosuppression*—this carries with it the severe risk of infection, which can be fatal in an already debilitated patient. At the moment there seems to be no easy solution to this; more specific suppression of the IR against allogeneic MHC Ags will be required.

Graft-vs-host reaction (GvH) This reaction occurs when competent lymphocytes are transferred to an immuno*in*competent recipient; the immunocompetent 'grafted cells' then regard the host cells as foreign and, in effect, reject the host, who, being immunoincompetent, cannot mount an IR against the graft. Such a situation can occur in medical practice when patients with *acute leukaemia, aplastic anaemia,* or *severe combined immunodeficiency disease* are given *bone marrow transplants.* These operations are usually restricted to transplants between MHC identical **siblings** (= children of the same parents), but GvH can still occur, suggesting that non-MHC genetic factors are involved. The reaction, when it occurs, consists of proliferation of graft lymphoid cells in the host's bone marrow, lymph nodes and spleen, after which they mount an attack on host tissue. The major mechanism is T-cell cytotoxicity, but humoral attack can contribute to the damage, which is widespread and frequently fatal.

IMMUNODEFICIENCY

Immunodeficiency is a defective functioning of any part of the immune system; this could be **primary**, as in congenital failure of development of certain facets of the system, or **secondary** to some other disease process. Deficiencies can occur in the specific immune mechanisms (T- or B-cell defects), or in components of the non-specific immune system (phagocytosis and complement).

Complement deficiencies Hereditary deficiencies are extremely rare, only a handful of cases having been recorded for most components; deficiencies of C9, C1q and components unique to the alternative pathway have not been found. The effects of the deficiency vary according to the component missing: lack of C3 can be fatal, since it represents the crux of the whole system, to which and from which everything leads; lack of later components is usually less severe but susceptibility to certain infections may be increased.

Complement deficiency can also be secondary to conditions in which there is continual C activation—e.g. SLE, due to the high levels of C fixing immune complexes.

Disorders of phagocytosis Several rare conditions occur in which the ability to kill ingested organisms is severely impaired; most of these involve the loss of an enzyme essential to the killing mechanism. Increased susceptibility to certain infections, some of which can be fatal, results.

T-cell deficiency This can readily be induced in experimental animals by **neonatal thymectomy** (*−ectomy* = cutting out), which results in a total loss of T-cells in the adult animal and hence absent cellular responses and impaired humoral responses to T-dependent Ag. The same effects are seen in the congenital condition, **thymic hypoplasia (Di George syndrome)**, in humans, in which embryological development of the thymus fails completely or partially. Affected individuals suffer from infections by organisms against which the main form of defence is a cellular response—viruses, intracellular bacteria (*Mycobacterium tuberculosis*), fungi, and protozoa. Treatment involves implanting a thymus, or administering thymus extracts or purified thymic hormones essential for T-cell development.

B-cell deficiencies In birds this can be produced by *neonatal bursectomy*; it is more difficult to induce in mammals, since there is no similarly distinct anatomical site for B-cell maturation. Several diseases occur in humans in which there are deficiencies in B-cell maturation resulting in failure to produce Ab and hence a-/hypogammaglobulinaemia (absent or lowered serum Ig).

Bruton's agammaglobulinaemia An hereditary (sex-linked) condition: serum Ig levels are low or non-existent, circulating B-cells are absent, and lymph nodes lack plasma cells. Children with the disease show recurrent infections with extracellular bacteria; nowadays, with antibiotics, very early death is prevented, but they frequently succumb to chronic respiratory infections. The most important part of treatment is to give human immune serum globulin, which contains Abs to common environmental pathogens and so confers passive immunity.

Common variable immunodeficiency A group of disorders, all characterized by hypogammaglobu-linaemia, but with each disorder having unique features as well. Not all Ig classes may be affected and some patients will also have a T-cell deficiency. Genetic factors may be involved but in some cases the defect appears to be acquired.

In addition to those diseases affecting *either* the humoral or the cellular IR there are a few which disrupt both aspects of the immune system. The most important of these is:

Severe combined immunodeficiency (Swiss type agammaglobulinaemia) Normal cellular and Ab responses are absent; the infants rarely survive more than a year or two because they are afflicted with acute and chronic infections by all microbial organisms. The defect lies at the lymphocyte stem cell level, so both B- and T-cells are missing. There is little effective treatment available at present for this condition. Bone marrow transplants (from a histocompatible donor) have been successful in only very rare cases and survival may be short-lived.

Currently making headlines in the media—and even achieving the status of a *TIME* 'cover story'—is a newly recognized immunodeficiency: **AIDS** (= **Acquired Immune Deficiency Syndrome**), which is manifested by a complete collapse of immunity. Apart from the fact that it is more prevalent in homosexual males and, to a much lesser extent, in self-injecting drug addicts and persons receiving repeated injections of plasma products—e.g. haemophiliacs, little is known about the disease. Death from recurring infection, or a rare form of cancer (Kaposi's sarcoma) is a common termination of AIDS.

HYPERGAMMAGLOBULINAEMIA

The term **hypergammaglobulinaemia** (*hyper* = too much; *gammaglobulin* = Ig; *aemia* = in the blood) covers a multitude of conditions in which there are raised levels of Ig in the serum. While high levels are found in chronic infections, the term is applied to those cases where they are a feature of the primary disease process.

Multiple myeloma (*multiple* = numerous or widespread; *myel* = bone marrow; *oma* = tumour): also known as **monoclonal gammopathy** (= a disturbance in Ig synthesis affecting only one clone). The condition is characterized by the uncontrolled proliferation, from one errant B-cell, of a single genetic clone of B-cells, with subsequent development into plasma cells all secreting Ig of identical class, subclass, specificity, etc.—therefore, **monoclonal (M) protein**. In 60% of cases IgG is the class of Ig produced (in accordance with its relative abundance in the serum): 30% of cases involve IgA, with rare examples of IgD and IgE being affected. Excessive IgM production is classified separately and termed **macroglobulinaemia**. In multiple myeloma, serum Igs with Ab specificities other than that of the myeloma become depressed, as the proliferating cells take over the bone marrow — the result is increased susceptibility to infection. Often, *free L chains*, produced in excess by the proliferating myeloma, appear in the urine and are called **Bence-Jones protein**; in some cases these Bence-Jones proteins can be seen in the urine in absence of a serum M protein.

Waldenström's macroglobulinaemia A condition in which proliferating cells produce excess IgM. The cells resemble both lymphocytes and plasma cells. The raised IgM levels considerably increase serum protein concentration and the viscosity of the blood. This can lead to decreased blood flow, which in turn can produce visual disturbances, muscle weakness and, if severe, cardiac failure and strokes.

Heavy-chain disease A rare condition involving the excess production of α, γ or μ heavy chains (in that order of frequency). These H chains seem to be abnormal and incapable of combining with L chains and so appear alone in the plasma.

Treatment

Treatment of these diseases involves: supportive measures to reverse the anaemia and combat infections; cytotoxic drugs to hit the dividing cells; if the hyperviscosity is severe, it may be necessary to remove the plasma and filter out the excess protein — **plasmapheresis** (*aphairesis* = withdrawal).

Epilogue

Biological science—like the life processes it seeks to fathom—is in a constant state of evolution. Consequently, a scientific book—like the runner who is constantly halving the distance between himself and an opponent—is furiously racing to catch up with its evolving science, but, inevitably, must always lag some fraction of a pace behind.

In *The Chain of Immunology*, our route map to the science of immunology, we hope that, at the time of going to press, our directions, signposts and descriptions are almost apace with the ever-changing immunological landscape—and reasonably free of misdirections.

But, above all, we remain hopeful that the reader will agree that *The Chain* has provided him with an intelligible guide to immunology. Though he recognizes that, as we warned at the outset, it does not aim to—indeed, cannot—tell him all about everything immunological, the reader will feel he has acquired a fair idea of what Nature was about when it saw fit to develop an adaptive immune system for its higher creatures.

If the reader comes away feeling better equipped to find his way around immunology, our immuno-cartographical (= map-making) mission will have been accomplished.

Bibliography for Extended Reading

Roitt I.M. (1980) *Essential Immunology*, 4e. Blackwell Scientific Publications, Oxford.

Fudenberg H.H. *et al* (1980) *Basic and Clinical Immunology*, 3e. Lange Medical Publications, Los Altos.

McConnell I. *et al* (1981) *The Immune System*, 2e. Blackwell Scientific Publications, Oxford.

Benacerraf B. & Unanue E.R. (1979) *Textbook of Immunology*, Williams & Wilkins, Baltimore.

Hudson L. & Hay F.C. (1980) *Practical Immunology*, 2e. Blackwell Scientific Publications, Oxford.

Index

A blood group substance 36
Ab *see* Antibody
ABO blood system 36–7
    antigens 36
Acquired immune deficiency
        syndrome 41
Adenosine triphosphate 6
Adjuvant 18, 38
Agammaglobulinaemia
    Bruton's 41
    Swiss Type 41
Agranulocytosis 36
AIDS 41
Alleles 8
    heterozygous 8
    homozygous 8
Allelic exclusion 8
Alloantigens 19
Allogeneic strains 8
Allotypes, immunoglobulins 13
Alum-precipitated antigen 18
Amidopyrine, reaction 36
Anaemia, and drug reactions 36
Anamnestic response 25
Anaphylactic degranulation 27
Anaphylaxis 34–5
    atopy 35
    bradykinin 35
    eosinophil chemotactic factor 35
    general symptoms 35
    histamine 34
    hyposensitization 35
    5-hydroxytryptamine 34
    and IgE 28
    leukotrienes 35
    neutrophil chemotactic factor 35
    passive cutaneous 27, 31
    pinnal 32
    platelet activating factor 35
    prostaglandins 34–5
    slow reacting substance (SRS-A) 35
Anaphylotoxin 13
    inactivator 14
Antibody(ies)
    affinity 20
    antinuclear 39
    blocking 35
    definition 2
    -dependent cell-mediated cytotoxicity
        (ADCC) 10, 27, 35
    monoclonal 32

Antigen 18–21
    accessible 6
    adjuvant 18
    anatomy 19
    /antibody binding 19
    characteristics 18–19
    chemical configuration 19
    chemical nature 18
    conjugated 18
    contact 18
    at critical period 22
    cross reactions 20
    definition 2, 3
    fate of 21
    foreignness 19
    hydrogen bonding 19–20
    immune tolerance 23
    infection 18
    ingestion 18
    inhalation 18
    injection 18
    ionic strength 19
    particulate 21
    routes of entry 18
    sequestered 19
    soluble 21
    synthetic 18
    T-dependent 23
    transplantation 18
    see also Self and Non-self
Antihistamines 35
Anti-lymphocyte globulin 23
Anti-lymphocyte serum 22–3, 40
Antinuclear antibody (ANA) 39
Antiserum, definition 2
Arthus reaction 37
Asthma 35
Atopy 35
Autoallergy 17
Autoimmune
    disease 38
    haemolytic anaemia 36
    thyroiditis 38
    treatment 39
Autoimmunity 17, 38–9
Azathioprine 40

B-cells 9, 15, 16
    activation, mechanisms 24
    Ag receptor 23

characteristics and functions 15
    deficiencies 40, 41
    gene expression 7
    memory 24
    pathway 23
    sub-sets 9
    -T-cell cooperation 23–4
B blood group substance 36
Bacillus Calmette-Guérin (BCG) 18,
        38
Basophils 10
    binding 28
Bence-Jones protein 41
Bird fancier's lung 37
Blast cells 6, 23
    transformation 23
Blood 9–15
    crossmatching 36–7
    groups 9, 36–7
    transfusion reaction 36
Booster dose (response) 25
Bordetella pertussis 18
Bradykinin, properties and actions 35
Bronchial-associated lymphoid tissue
        (BALT) 16
Bruton's agammaglobulinaemia 41, 42
Bursa of Fabricius 15

Cell
    activities 6–8
    anatomy 4–6
    division 6
    function 3–4
    membrane 6
        antigens 15
Cellular
    immune response 28–9
        effector T-cells 28
        lymphokines 28, 29
            functions 29
        self-restriction 28
Centriole 5, 6
Centromere 4
Chemotaxis 9
Chromatid
    definition 4
    separation 6
Chromatin, definition 4
Chromosome, definition 4
Circulating immune complex 37

Cirrhosis, primary biliary 39
Clone (clonal) 23
    deletion 38
    expansion 23
    inactivation 38
    selection hypothesis of Burnet 25
Co-dominance, genes 8
Complement 13–15
    barrage 13, 15
    Cl esterase inhibitor 15
    C3 13
        convertase 13–15
        C3a 13
        C3b 13
            inactivator 14
    cascade 13
    components 13
    control mechanisms 15
    deficiencies 40–1
    factors 13–14
    fixation test 31
    lysis test 31
    pathways, alternative, common and
        classical 13
    terminal end 11
Congenic strains 8
Constant domains 11
Constant regions 11
Contact sensitivity 38
Coomb's test 27
Corticosteroids in transplantation 40
Covert immune response see Immune
        response, covert
Crossmatching, blood 36–7
Cross reactions 20
Cyclosporin A 40
Cytoplasm 5
Cytoskeleton 5
Cytotoxic/cytolytic hypersensitivity
        35–6

Delayed hypersensitivity 15, 37–8, 38
Dendritic cell, role 21
Di George syndrome 41
Dinitrochlorobenzene (DNCB) 38
Diploid cells 4
Disseminated intravascular
        coagulation 36
Disulfide bridges 10
DNA, definition 4
Domains, definition, constant 2
    variable 2, 11
Donor, definition 2
Double diffusion technique 30
Drug
    -induced haemolytic anaemia 36
    reactions 36

Effector cells 23
Electrophoresis 10
Endoplasmic reticulum 5
    rough 5
    smooth 5

Endotoxins 18
Enzyme-linked immunosorbent assay
        (ELISA) 31
Eosinophil(s) 10
    chemotactic factor of anaphylaxis
        (ECF-A) 35
Epitope, definition 1
    -paratope binding 19
    size, heterogeneity and specificity 19
    shared 20–1
    similar 20
Erythrocytes in blood grouping 9, 36
Extrinsic allergic alveolitis 37

Fab 12
Farmer's lung 37
Fc fragment 12
    region of IgE 10
Foreignness 19
    degree 19–20
Fragments
    antigen-binding (Fab) 12
    crystallizable 12
    immunoglobulin 12
Freund's complete adjuvant 18, 38
Freund's incomplete adjuvant 18

Gametes 7
Gammaglobulins 10
Gammopathy, monoclonal 41
'Gatekeeper effect', IgE 28
Gene 8–9
    dominant 8
    expression 7
    function 8–9
    immune response (Ir) 22
    recessive 8
    repressed 7
Genetically related factor 21
Genotype 8
Germ cells, function 3
Germ-line theory 25
Glomerulonephritis 39
Golgi apparatus 5
Graft rejection 8, 17, 39–40
    patterns 40
Graft-vs-host disease 40
Granules 6
Granulocytes 10
Granuloma formation 18, 21
Graves' disease 38
Group O blood 36
    see also Blood groups
Gut-associated lymphoid tissue
        (GALT) 16

H substance 36
H-2 region 8–9
Haematopoietic tissue 9
Haemolytic disease of newborn 36
Haploid number of chromosomes 7
Hapten 18–19
Hay fever 35

Heavy chains
    amino-acid sequencing 11
    disease 42
    framework 11
    hinge regions 11, 27
    variable regions 11
Hinge region 11, 27
Histamine, action 34
Histocompatibility antigens 6, 8
Horror autotoxicus 19
Human leucocyte antigen 8–9
Humoral
    element 10
    immune response 25–6
        theory, instructive 25
            germ-line 25
            selective 25
            somatic mutation 25–6
    technology 29–32
    precipitation 29–32
Hybridization 32
Hybridoma technology 32
5-Hydroxytryptamine, action 34
Hypergammaglobulinaemia 41
Hypersensitivity 17, 34–6
    definition 2
    Type I 24, 34
    Type II (cytotoxic/cytolytic)
        35–6
        ADCC 35
        complement activation 35
        opsonization 35
    Type III (immune complex
        mediated) 37
    Type IV, delayed 15, 37–8, 38
Hyposensitization 35
Hypotension in anaphylaxis 35

Idiotypes, immunoglobulins 13
Immune
    competence 3
    complex mediated hypersensitivity
        37
    reaction, definition 1–2
    recognition, definition 1
    response, covert 2, 22–4
        definition 1
            cellular 1
            humoral 1
            primary 1
            secondary 1
        gene 22
        ontogeny 3
        overt, and immune reaction 2,
            25–33
            adoptive transfer 25
            cellular immune response 28–9
            humoral immune response
                25–8
            immunoglobulins M, G, A, D, E
                26–8
            immunotechnology 29–33

primary 25
secondary 25
phylogeny 3
tolerance 23
high zone 23
low zone 23
Immunity, definition 2
active 2
passive 2
Immunization, definition 2
Immunocompetence 22–3
Immunodeficiency 22, 40–1
acquired immune deficiency
syndrome (AIDS) 41
common variable 41
severe combined 41
Immunodiffusion techniques 29–30
double diffusion 30
Mancini technique 30
single radial 30
Immunoelectrophoresis 30–1
modifications 31
Immunofluorescence technique 31
Immunogen, definition 2
Immunoglobulin(s)
allotypes 13
classes 11
definition 10
disulfide bridges 10
fragments 12
genetic variants 12
heavy chains 10, 11
idiotypes 13
isotypes 12–13
light chains 10, 11–12
structure 10–11
sub-classes 11
Immunoglobulin A 27
J-chain 27
secretory 27
properties 27
serum 27
Immunoglobulin D 27–8
structure 28
Immunoglobulin E 28
anthelminthic action 28
properties 28
Immunoglobulin G 26–7
activation of classical pathway 26
agglutination of particulate Ag 27
heterocytotropic antibody 27
memory 26
neutralizes toxins and viruses 27
opsonin 27
placental transport 26
precipitation of soluble Ag 26–7
structure 26
Immunoglobulin M 26
in ABO system 36
affinity 26
J-chain 26
molecular weight 26

natural antibodies 26
structure 26
Immunological uniqueness 8
Immunology, definition 1, 2
Immunosuppression 22–3
biological 22–3
induction, chemical 22
radiological 22
surgical 23
Immunotechnology 29–33
cellular 33
humoral 29–32
hybridoma 32–3
monoclonal Abs 32–3
T-cell markers 32–3
Inbred strains 7, 8
Infection 17
Inflammation, definition 2
Interferon 9, 29
Interleukins 23
Irradiation, lymphoid, total 40
Isoantibodies 19
Isoantigens 19
Isotypes, immunoglobulin 12–13

J-chain, IgA 27

K (Killer) cell 9, 10
Kaposi's sarcoma 41
Konglutinin activating factor
(KAF) 14

Labelled Ab immunotechniques 31
LADs 9, 39
Langerhans cells 17, 21
Large granular lymphocytes 9
Large pyroninophilic cell 6, 23
LATS 38
Leucocytes 9
Leukotrienes 35
Leu system 32
Light chains, Ig 10, 11–12
kappa 12
lambda 12
paratope 12
variable region 11
Locus 8
Long acting thyroid stimulator
(LATS) 38
Lymph nodes 16
structure 16
Lymphocytes 9
activated 9
activating determinants 9, 39
adopted transfer 25
mixed reaction 33
in specific IR 21
stimulation 23–4
clonal expansion 23
mitosis 23
T- and B-cells 23
T-independence 24
transformation 23

traffic 16–17
transformation test 33
Lymphoid
follicles 16
irradiation, total 40
tissues 15–17
central 15
secondary 16
Lymphokines 28, 37
interferon 29
lymphotoxin 29
macrophage, chemotactic factor 29
migration inhibition factor 29
mitogenic factor 29
skin reactive factor 29
Lymphotoxin 29
Lysosomes 5, 10
Ly system 32

Macroglobulinaemia 41
Waldenström's 42
Macrophage 10
activating factor 29
chemotactic factor 29
migration inhibition factor 29
test 33
role 21
and T-cell pathway 23
Major histocompatibility complex 8
antigens 8–9
restriction 21
Mancini technique 30
Mast cells 17
binding 28
Maturation, immunological 3
Mediators 10
vasoactive, release 28
Meiosis, definition 7
Membrane attack mechanism 15
Memory, definition 1
Messenger RNA 4
MHC see Major histocompatibility
complex
Microphage 10
Migration inhibition test, macrophage
29, 33
Mitochondria 5
Mitogenic factor 29
Mitotic spindle 6
Mixed lymphocyte reaction 9, 33
Monoclonal
Abs 32
gammopathy 41
(M)protein 41
Monocyte 9–10
Mononuclear
cells 9
phagocyte system 17
mRNA, definition 4
Multicellular organism, function 3
Multiple myeloma 41
Mutation 7–8

Myasthenia gravis 38
Mycobacterium tuberculosis 38
Myeloma, multiple 41

N-terminal end 11
Natural killer cell 9
Neuromuscular junction 38
Neutrophil
   chemotactic factor of anaphylaxis
      (NCF-A) 35
   in specific IR 21
Non-lymphoid tissues 17
Non-self 19
   acceptance 22
   histocompatibility antigens 8
Nuclear envelope 4
Nucleolus, definition 4
Nucleotide, definition 4
Nucleus, definition 4
Null cells 9

Oedema and hypersensitivity 34
OKT system 32
Opsonin 27
Opsonization 35
Organ transplantation 39–40
Organelles 5
Ouchterlony technique 30
Overt immune response and immune
      reaction 25–33
   see also Immune response, overt

Papain, action 12
Paratope, definition 1
Passive
   cutaneous anaphylaxis 27, 31
   sensitization 27
Pepsin, action 12
Perigranular membrane 10
Phagocytosis 10
   disorders 41
Phagosome 5
Phenacetin, reaction 36
Phenotype 8
Picryl chloride 38
Pinnal anaphylaxis 32
Pinocytosis 10
Plasma cell 16, 23
Plasmapheresis 42
Platelet 10
   activating factor 35
   aggregation 36
Polymorphonuclear cells (polymorphs)
   10

Polysome 5
Precipitation techniques 29–32
Prednisone, in transplantation 40
Prostaglandins, properties and actions
      34–5
Protein
   Bence-Jones 41
   M (monoclonal) 41
Purified protein derivative(PPD) 38

Radioimmunoassay 31
Reagin 28
Receptor
   antigen, T- and B-cells 23
   definition 1, 6
   recognition 9
Recognition
   definition 1
   receptors 9
Red blood cells *see* Erythrocytes
Reticuloendothelial system 17
Reticuloepithelial system 17
Rhesus
   incompatibility 35
   system, antigens 36–7
Rheumatoid arthritis 39
Ribosomal RNA 4, 6
Ribosome 5
Rosettes 15
rRNA 4

Secretory vacuoles 5
Sedormid, reaction 36
Self, histocompatibility antigens 8
Sensitivity, contact 38
Sensitization
   definition 2
   passive 27
Serological determination 9
Serum sickness 37
Sessile macrophage 17
Single radial immunodiffusion 30
Skin reactive factor 29
Slow reacting substance of anaphylaxis
      (SRS-A) 35
Somatic
   cells, function 3–4
   mutation theory 25
Specificity, definition 1
Spleen 16
Stem cells 9
Suicide cell 10
Suppressor T-cells 38
Surface markers 6

Swiss type agammaglobulinaemia 41
Syngeneic strains 7, 8
Systemic lupus erythematosus 39

T-cells 9
   Ag receptor 23
   characteristics and functions 15,
      16
   cytotoxic 15, 28, 40
   deficiency 40, 41
   gene expression 7
   helper 15, 28
   markers 32–3
   pathway 23
   primed 37
   sub-sets 9, 15, 28
   suppressor 15, 28, 38
Target tissues 17
Template hypotheses, direct and
      indirect 25
Thrombocyte 10
   see also Platelet
Thymectomy, neonatal 41
Thymic
   hypoplasia (Di George syndrome)
      22, 41
   leukaemia antigen 15
Thymidine nucleoside 7
Thymine, DNA specific 4, 7
Thymus 15
Thyroiditis, autoimmune 38
Thyrotoxicosis 38
Tissue typing 39
Total lymphoid irradiation 40
Transfer RNA 5
Transplantation
   antigens 8
   organ 39–40
Tuberculin test 38
Tumour surveillance 17
Twins, identical 7, 8

Universal recipients 36
Urticaria 35

Vasoactive mediators, release 28

Waldenström's macroglobulinaemia
   42
Wheal and flare reaction 34
White blood cells and tumour
      surveillance 17

Xenogeneic strains 8